I0879994

PENGUIN BOOKS

THREADING WORLDS: CONVERSATIONS ON MENTAL HEALTH

SINGAPORE AND MENTAL HEALTH

As an internationally recognised spiritual teacher, professional artist, social healer, life coach, and community leader, Hun Ming Kwang is relentless in his mission to illuminate individuals to their deepest truths, callings and authentic selves, helping them awaken and harness their power to actualize their lives at their highest creative potential. Today, he has helped over 10,000 individuals transform their lives and attain a higher level of awareness.

He also focuses on championing humanitarian campaigns and efforts to invoke and inspire awareness on social causes such as mental health and suicide prevention at a national level. He is the founder and co-artistic director of ThisConnect.today, where he designs and produces experiential art, interactive films and conscious conversations to make a difference to the public.

OTHER BOOKS IN THE SERIES

Stories We Don't Tell, Penguin Random House SEA, 2022
Growing Pains, Penguin Random House SEA, 2022
Weaving between Light and Shadows, Said and Unsaid,
Penguin Random House SEA, 2022

Threading Worlds:
Conversations on Mental Health

Singapore and Mental Health

Hun Ming Kwang

PENGUIN BOOKS

An imprint of Penguin Random House

PENGUIN BOOKS

USA | Canada | UK | Ireland | Australia
New Zealand | India | South Africa | China | Southeast Asia

Penguin Books is part of the Penguin Random House group of companies whose addresses can be found at global.penguinrandomhouse.com

Published by Penguin Random House SEA Pvt. Ltd
9, Changi South Street 3, Level 08-01,
Singapore 486361

Penguin Random House SEA

First published in Penguin Books by Penguin Random House SEA 2022

10 9 8 7 6 5 4 3 2 1

ISBN 9789815058277

Typeset in Garamond by MAP Systems, Bengaluru, India

www.penguin.sg

Contents

Foreword

The latest Singapore Mental Health Study shows one in seven people has experienced some mental health challenges in their lifetime and more than seventy-five per cent of these did not seek any professional help.[1] *Threading Worlds: Conversations on Mental Health* Volumes seek to close this treatment gap.

The transcribed authentic voices of healthcare professionals and other community leaders and those with lived experiences will help us reach the self-realization of our own state of mental wellness. It will move us to co-create a safe space for the community to talk openly about the challenges and the solutions with courage and empathy.

One of the causes of the treatment gap is the stigmatization of the condition, driving us away from seeking treatment. I have been to ThisConnect's multimedia art exhibitions and one of the works—*Connection without Sight* shows us how we can connect deeply through our primal senses and emotional centres without succumbing to the superficial judgement of sight.

---

[1] Subramaniam, M., E. Abdin, J. A. Vaingankar, S. Shafie, B. Y. Chua, R. Sambasivam, Y. J. Zhang, et al., 'Tracking the Mental Health of a Nation: Prevalence and Correlates of Mental Disorders in the Second Singapore Mental Health Study', Epidemiology and Psychiatric Sciences 29, 2020: e29. doi:10.1017/S2045796019000179

Active listening is essential for deep understanding with empathy without which the advice we give and receive are likely to be irrelevant and superfluous. Another work—*I Feel You* will enable us to stand in the shoes of others and be there to hold that safe sacred space for another human being.

Masks of Singapore, a six-month local community self-awareness mask-making project, depict the façade that most people portray to one another in our daily interactions. We wear these 'masks' to suppress our true mental state. The making of masks will help us discover our true self and give ourselves permission to express our truth more freely than ever.

This project is a cool way to create a healing place for us to courageously confront our own mental health challenges in a safe space. Wherever these books are found, a safe space is created to mine the comprehensive information leading one to seek treatment. I wish Ming Kwang and his team luck and may their endeavours be perfectly accomplished.

Dr William Wan, PhD, JP.
General Secretary,
Singapore Kindness Movement

To You: A Message From The Author

Dear Reader,

If by a stroke of luck, a gesture of goodwill, something about this book resonated with you, it found its way to you, and landed in your hands—let it be a sign that there are certain answers in your life that you're searching for.

Before we begin, I would like to invite you to take a moment to picture this:

You're a student in your teens or early twenties. You're spending thousands of dollars on a formal education as you work your way up to a university degree, studying subjects only for the purpose of excelling in the exams, while juggling several other commitments such as an internship, a part-time job, an extra-curricular activity, to boost your credentials and show your potential employers that you have some degree of holistic development, real-world experience, and a life outside of your studies. Along the way, you might have countless nights of overwhelming stress, pressure, burnout, and negative downward spirals. You ask yourself endlessly: are you disappointing your family? Are you failing the expectations that others have of you? Are you on track to landing a stable job once you graduate? Do you have enough commitments on your plate to ensure you're not any less ambitious than your peers? Your teachers might have good intentions, but the most they tell you is 'Don't stress too much, just remain calm, be positive, be happy, and do your best'—as if those things never automatically occurred to you before. In a world full of adults who appear to have figured out all the answers to life, are you a failure if you can't be positive and calm without distracting yourself and numbing away your anger, sadness, and negativity?

This might also be the period where you struggle to make sense and find your place in your social world. How do people view you? Who are the friends who are going to stick by you as you enter adulthood and into the working world? Who are the people you need to be networking with so that you can position yourself favourably? If you don't manage to find a life partner now, will you still have the time and opportunities to do so once the rat race begins? Are you considered a failure if you never end up settling down with a partner and starting a family?

Or, perhaps you're a corporate executive or a full-time employee in your mid-twenties to thirties, working your daily nine-to-five job. When you first started out, you might have felt excited and driven to finally leave your mark on the world and fulfil your ambitions. But a couple of years later, your life has been entirely segmented into three parts: your day job, the couple of hours at night you have to rest before the next day, and the weekend, where you attempt to make up for all the rest, recreational activities, or social needs that you missed out during the week. Your job pays the bills, but it becomes a mechanical task for you to get through every day. It might not necessarily challenge you to grow as a person. It might not fulfil you, or it might not even be something in your interest in the first place—but you had no choice but to take it on anyway because the job market was bad, there was pressure on you to be doing something great with your life as a culmination of everything you've learnt after you graduated, and you spent nearly twenty years of your life studying and working relentlessly for a paper degree that only serves to tell your potential employers that you're knowledgeable and a specialist in that particular field of study. Surely you've got to work a job that justifies the amount of money, time, blood, sweat, and tears spent on your formal education at the expense of other pursuits that might be less lucrative, but more fulfilling! Otherwise, what did you give up your dreams for? And the unfortunate thing is, perhaps by the fifth year of your career, you're wondering if it is time to switch jobs or try your hands at something new. And for a while, it does bring a breath of fresh air into your life, but after a period of time, you find yourself back at the same spot again—stuck in an endless loop.

Perhaps you're a fifty-something veteran in your field, and you're looking for change, because you've gotten what you wanted out of your career and realized that there's something more you want out of your life. Perhaps you've realized that you neglected every other aspect of your life apart from your career, and you want to rectify that. Perhaps you're a seventy-something retiree, and you're wondering what else there is to life besides living it day by day as you wait for the day you die.

When you encounter such instances, when you question where your life is at, where it is going, what really matters to you, and what your purpose in life really is at the end of the day, I would like to assure you that it's a step you have taken towards looking inwards at yourself. And as much pain and struggle or joy and happiness as it may bring, **keep going**.

Sometimes, we give up our dreams and settle for less while telling ourselves that what we have is good enough. Sometimes, unfortunate circumstances happen to us and make us give up parts of ourselves. Sometimes, the life that we live does not belong to us, but to the expectations of us, to the intentions of others, and to the popular dreams that are trendy at the moment. We gather these second-hand dreams and ideas that belong to others and try to cobble together what our lives could be and what we desire. Be that as it may the answers don't lie there, but within us. However well and good our intentions are, in chasing after the lives of others, we reject and deny what is fundamentally at the root of ourselves: *ourselves.*

The term 'mental health' has rapidly gained traction over the last couple of years, especially in the wake of the pandemic, but there is still a large lack of understanding that mental health is a spectrum in which everyone has their own place depending on where they are in their journey. Some of us are battling mental health conditions and illnesses. Some of us are in the middle, where what we're going through is not necessarily deemed severe enough to be classified as an illness or disorder, but we feel the brunt of our symptoms nonetheless in our everyday lives, and it hinders us from thriving and performing at our optimum capabilities when we need to. Some of us are doing relatively well holistically in the different aspects of our lives, and we're looking at how to take it to the next level. Yet, as I say this, I want to emphasize that somebody who is thriving in their lives can absolutely still go through mental health struggles that are specific to their life's circumstances. Likewise, people who struggle chronically with mental illnesses or disorders can absolutely have days where they're feeling good. Essentially, everybody has mental health, and we relate to it in ways that are entirely unique to our circumstances, our psyche, and our history.

Where you fall on the spectrum is entirely unique to you, and that is why resolving your issues is not a matter of looking outwards at what people have done to resolve their issues and replicating that—although that can certainly give you more data and clarity on what works and what doesn't—but more importantly about looking inwards, understanding the true nature of the issue (since our external reality is really nothing more than a reflection of who

we are inside), and examining the core of who *you* are, so that you can do what *you* need to do to triumph over *your* challenges and live *your* **best** life.

Presently, the world is going through a mental health epidemic. More than ever, people are experiencing increasingly severe bouts of depression, anxiety, and on the most severe end of the spectrum, suicidal thoughts, suicide attempts, and suicide cases. In fact, I want to highlight this particular incident that stands out to me. In 2021, a sixteen-year-old student from River Valley High School in Singapore was charged with the murder of a thirteen-year-old schoolmate. Our hearts sank when the news was publicly released. He was found to have been previously assessed at the Institute of Mental Health (IMH) in 2019 after attempting suicide. I believe that this incident highlights the state that children and younger folk are in these days in terms of their mental health and overall wellbeing. There is much more to be done and ground to be covered as this incident happened despite the increase of mental health and wellness programmes in schools and workplaces.

It is precisely because of this that we need to tackle the whole issue of mental health not by adopting a blanket one-size-fits-all solution, but by looking inwards, because suicide never happens in a moment. It never ever does. There are a million moments leading up to that point. Each moment we choose not to face and deal with questions that matter to or bother us, emotions that are 'unpleasant', or conflicts and baggage in our lives, we risk falling or spiralling further down the spectrum. Our issues never really go away until we deal with them and resolve them at the root level head on.

Our life begins the moment we're born—especially in the moments we can no longer consciously remember. The very first time you opened your mouth and cried out loud as a baby, what were your parents' reactions? What was *your* response to that?

The very first time you displayed any bout of anger or rebellion, what were the reactions of the people around you? Did they talk down to you and reprimand you? Did your parents tell you that a good son or daughter would never have exhibited such behaviours? Were you present to the anger and the subtle shame and guilt that ran inside your programming? What did you learn about your emotions, social behaviours, and boundaries consequently from those incidents? The very first time you cried and wished you had your parents' approval and attention but was left waiting and wanting, what was *your* response to that? What did *you* tell yourself about love and relationships?

The very first time you opened up to a teacher or a family member about your dreams to be an artist, a singer, an astronaut, a designer, what was their response? What was *your* response as a reaction to that? What did *you* tell yourself about dreams and reality? What were *your* notions and beliefs around success?

Perhaps, this is about your identity. The very first time you realized that you fell somewhere on the LGBTQ spectrum, and you didn't exactly turn out exactly the way your parents or society expected you to be—'normal'—and you chose courage, came out to these people, but were rejected, or the first time you witnessed someone else in a similar boat get rejected and judged by others, what did it teach *you* about family? What did *you* tell yourself about *your* identity? What did *you* tell yourself about courage, and how did it shape your relationship with it?

One of the most common myths we have around pain is that time heals all wounds, but that couldn't be further from the truth. Time makes us forget that those wounds exist in the first place—it gives us the opportunity to evade or numb ourselves with drugs, alcohol, entertainment, or some other form of escapism from our pain, until we forget about them. And sometimes we go into a delusion thinking that these issues are no more. Silly us.

It doesn't matter what the topic is—the very first statements we tell ourselves about that topic, grows with us as we grow as people throughout the various stages of our lives, and they get reinforced over time as we encounter similar incidents repeatedly. And oftentimes, while these statements may have served and saved us from pain once upon a time in the very first moment, they tend to do us more harm than good in the long run. For instance, if you've always been told that crying is bad and you were punished for it, you might have resorted to numbing away any nuance of sadness or grief the moment you feel it. Doing that might have saved you punishment from your parents while growing up, but as an adult, that numbing has its own repercussions. You might become so numb and disconnected from yourself that you can't tell what matters to you anymore, and you're always looking outwards for answers. Each time you suppress an emotion just adds another drop into the pressure cooker of emotions inside you that's bubbling and waiting to explode when you least expect it, and when you're least prepared to deal with it.

Emotions have always been a tricky topic that we've not yet managed to successfully incorporate well into our upbringing at home and in the education system. Our understanding of emotions is largely limited to happiness, anger, and sadness, but what about everything else in between? What about the subtle emotions like guilt, jealousy, shame, disgust, contempt, or envy? Not to point fingers at anyone in particular, as most parents and educators are only teaching what they've been taught and what they know, and we simply do not know any better, but some of the most unhelpful advice given to kids in school regarding emotions is to just 'not be sad because it doesn't help' and 'be positive and things will work out'. What we've gotten out of that advice are generations of people who are completely out of touch with their emotions, particularly those that are deemed as 'difficult and unpleasant', and are going through the motions of their lives without ever fully participating, engaging, and involving *themselves* in how it unfolds. This only serves to worsen the mental health struggles we face and potentially turn them into long-term mental health disorders.

The unconventional wisdom is to be able to receive the pain such that the pain completes its course. And when the pain no longer has a reason to make you suffer, then perhaps it's time for you to heal. And if you are not busy dying, maybe you will expend some energy into what it takes to live. And if you live, the next question is, how alive do you want to be?

It is crucial to understand that having the ability to manage our emotions is tantamount to managing ourselves as people who are functional and able to contribute value meaningfully to society. It is integral to be able to deal with crisis situations, to being able to lead and work with a team of people from all walks of life with various personalities. It is necessary to be able to connect with another person on a deeper level and hear the things that are left unsaid. It is absolutely paramount to maintaining a healthy overall wellbeing, because a heavy suppression of our emotions eventually leads to the damage on our physical body that manifests as various forms of diseases and illnesses.

The repercussions and consequences of not being able to deal with crisis, of not being able to deal with people both in our personal and professional lives, of having our emotional baggage manifest itself as physical diseases such as cancers, diabetes, or even autoimmune diseases can leave a deep negative impact that takes us years to recover from. Some people never really quite recover. Some resign to the fact that their life is filled with woes so much so that they have accepted that this is where and how their lives end, and these are the people who unfortunately never come to the awareness that there is a way out.

I want to say this: **There is always a way out, no matter how bad circumstances present themselves to you**.

Fortunately, if you're finding *yourself* and looking for *your* place in this world, there is a way—your mental and emotional health is a starting point from which you can begin looking into your psyche, your past, your present, how your future will play out, and what you can do NOW to shape them—just as you shape your life, your paths, and your destinies.

Threading Worlds: Conversations on Mental Health is a literary compilation of conversations my team and I had with seventy-five other contributors in Singapore from March 2021 to May 2021 around the topic of mental health and emotional wellness. These seventy-five contributors come from all walks of life—doctors, nurses, caregivers, counsellors, psychiatrists, therapists, policymakers, social workers, politicians, business leaders, coaches, and youths—and we had facilitated conversations with them on their perspectives on the mental health scene, their own personal journeys, as well as what needs to be done at an individual, community, and national level so that we can move forward and evolve as a collective. Each conversation was transcribed word-for-word with minimized filters deliberately to retain the essence of each conversation such that readers are able to immerse themselves in the conversation and experience it as though they were present in the very moment when the conversation first took place.

This book is intended to serve as a mental and emotional health literacy resource worldwide, and especially in countries like Japan, Korea, and Thailand, where suicide rates are the highest, and the third-world countries where looking inwards and the whole idea of mental health is a luxury in relation to the survivalist fights they have to battle each day instead. Through the perspectives from different walks of life, stories of vulnerability and journeys of recovering and rediscovering oneself, instead of telling people what mental health is and what it is not, we aim to create an immersive experience that allows you to connect to yourself and derive the personal wisdoms and lessons embedded within these stories with your inner-knowing that you can apply to your life. It is best experienced in a distraction-free state when you are able to be *fully and wholly present to yourself* as you experience the book.

As much as you are able to at this moment in your life, I would like to invite you to begin approaching this not exclusively as a mental-health-specific topic, but as a journey of illumination that you embark on to seek the important answers to the questions you have about yourself, your life, and the world around you, so that you can find your footing and live a life that truly matters to you at the end of the day. Many of us, at some point in our lives, ask the bigger questions with heavier weights: Who am I? Where did I come from? What am I meant to do? What is my purpose? What is my truest self? What is the meaning of life itself? And what about my life? How do I live a worthwhile life?

That is right. This has always been about your life, not just your mental health. When we run so hard trying to find our way out of the overwhelming barrage of circumstances our lives are presented with, we might find ourselves reaching our breaking point and collapsing physically, mentally, emotionally, even spiritually. At times when we are defeated, there is no way upwards but to muster every drop of willpower in us to crawl our way to the door and roll ourselves out.

We live in a world where our actions create a ripple effect down the road. Consequently, there are the forces of cause and effect in play. What matters is not what happens in the past or the future, but what you choose to do right now that consequently affects the trajectory of your life. Every passing moment is a second chance to turn it all around. As the saying goes: 'It is easier to build strong children than to repair broken men.' For us to nurture a generation free from the weight of the pain that we and our ancestors bear, we must first heal ourselves to break out of the chains that bind us. To find ourselves, we must first have the courage to give up what we believe is the truth about ourselves and walk the path of self-discovery. Only then do we know what it takes to make a difference to ourselves, and can we have the power to teach others what it means to be a human being in their own right, and be that beacon of light to those finding their way out of the dark.

Ultimately, my goal is to see a society where people thrive, not just survive, and are empowered to be bold, be free, and be ourselves. To have a conscious connection, not just with another person, but with ourselves. To embark on a journey to seek the answers we're searching for. To dare to dream, and dare to make those dreams happen. To gather our courage and take leaps of faith, even if we don't know where and how we'll land. To confront our deepest fears. To stand on the roof and declare our deepest truths to the world. To strike a pose and shout out to the universe, 'This is Me!' To challenge our adversities. To fail in our quest to live a good and fulfilling life, because it is through those failures that we learn what it means to stand for something that matters to us, time and time again, against all odds. To feel deeply, love deeply, and know that there is absolutely no shame in expressing ourselves authentically, no matter what people think.

One life saved can save many other lives. When we embark on the journey of living a life that truly matters to us, we also empower ourselves to step onto a path that enables us to touch another person's life with our highest being. A path along which we create a future that we're excited to step into, a path where we *leave our mark* on the world—so that when the time comes for us to go, we will go not with regrets, but with the knowledge that we have given every drop of our tears, sweat, and blood to living a life true to ourselves.

All of us are a walking morass of questions, on the journey of seeking the answers to living fully alive, and enjoying the ride along the way. Again, to reiterate what I said in the beginning—if by the stroke of luck, a gesture of goodwill, something about this book resonated with you, found its way to you, and landed in your hands—let it be a sign that there are certain answers in your life that you're searching for, and may this book contain some of the lessons and wisdom that can empower you on this journey. When you are done, pass it to another person to pay it forward. Because you never know who may need just that ounce of light to get themselves back on track, since we have adapted to become experts in masking our emotions (I say this sarcastically . . . but this is a very real issue today).

I share this message from a space of love and courage, as somebody who has taken a stand for the transformation of ourselves, transcendence of our limitations, and actualization of our innate potential. And when the time comes, I look forward to meeting you, the reader of this book, someday—the parts of you that can be a beacon of light to the higher consciousness of this world. May our stories, journeys, and collective wisdoms and transformations inspire even more people to begin looking into themselves so that they can begin their own journey of transformation, so that they live their marks on this world, so that when the time comes for us to go, we will go not with regrets, but with the spirit of the life that we've lived well with dignity.

Hun Ming Kwang
Founder, Creative Director, Author of ThisConnect.today

SPECIAL CHAPTER

'There Is No Deadline for Grief'

By Hun Ming Kwang

Among the spectrum of emotions available to us, grief lies at the deeper end. It is an overwhelming, intense form of sadness, coupled with a myriad of deep emotions that fundamentally stems from loss.

One of the biggest misconceptions we have in approaching grief, and pain, is that *time heals all wounds.* This misconception happens not only to individuals, but can be seen across our society where things are constantly moving forward at a relentless pace, regardless of one's state of being. For example, when we suffer a deep loss, such as the death of our loved ones, we usually take a period of compassionate leave from work to plan the wake and funeral and handle the legal administrative paperwork. Once the funeral is over, we get back to the office and life goes on. The underlying assumption in this is that we can put a timeline to grief. We have a cultural belief that at the end of three to five days of the wake and the funeral, it will be time again for us to get back to the grind and return to our jobs, because 'that is what everybody does and it is normal to do so', even if we feel emotionally incomplete.

Similarly, here's another misconception about grief—that it only happens when we experience death.

What many people don't realize is that grief comes in many forms, particularly during times of change. We can grieve the loss of a loved one—during a romantic breakup, the end of a friendship, the divorce of our parents, and even when one of our family members move out and away from home. We can grieve the loss of a beloved job, the destruction of nature, the change in our environment where we used to feel a sense of belonging, safety and security. We can grieve the loss of independence, the loss of an opportunity, or the loss of hope for the future. We can grieve for the memories of childhood we longed for the moment we graduate from school, and when we realize the working world was not all it was made up to be. We can grieve for the dreams we have long given up on, feeling empty and at a loss in the knowledge that we've settled for less in life. We can also grieve during the happiest moments of our lives, wishing the moment would never end just so that we don't have to deal with a different side of reality.

There is a popular framework that tells us how to understand grief intellectually. This framework states that there are seven emotional stages to grief. It usually starts with shock or disbelief, followed by denial, anger, bargaining or justifying, guilt or depression, then acceptance or hope. From this framework alone, we can gather that grief comes with a myriad of emotions. Of these, the most commonly recognized stages are the ones where we withdraw ourselves or express our sorrows in tears. The stages of grief are not isolated to emotional ones alone. Grief can have a physical effect on our body and health, as well as on our physical space and environment, changing the state of social settings. This is a basic understanding of what grief is, as I've come to know, working with people from all walks of life in the last decade. However, I found it to be true, even for myself, that what most people struggle most with is unpacking the difficult complex emotions that come with grief. Understandably so, since most of us grew up in an environment where emotional literacy was never emphasized, or taught to us.

The layman's definition of emotions may revolve around happy, sad and angry, which are by nature more recognizable as they are more obviously expressed and can be detected easily. Grief, however, is an extreme form of sadness, more subtle, sometimes described as 'a black hole in the heart'. Many of us just simply do not know how to deal with an emotion that affects a person at such depth. There are times where the hole feels like there is no end to it. Oftentimes, we only realize the extent to which we have been affected by grief at a much later stage, usually when our physical or mental health deteriorates quite severely. This is why it is important to raise awareness about what grief truly is.

We must first establish that everyone experiences grief in deeply personal and different ways. No two people grieve the same way. Some grieve by mourning openly, others by mourning privately. Some grieve by talking about the people that have passed or the loss that they've experienced, while others prefer not to talk about it at all and to deal with it themselves. Some seek comfort in religion and their social circles, while others question their faith or spirituality. In any case, I feel it is about respecting the individual's choice. This chapter does not serve to tell people what is right or wrong. It only serves to give people the awareness and the clarity to put to words the states that they are dealing with, so that they can begin to make a more conscious choice about how they would like to move forward in their lives.

The process of grieving can look frightening, one that involves leaving behind something that was so integral to our lives. Grieving is also hard when we spend some amount of energy, resources or time to form deep relationships or even simple attachments, and it doesn't work out.

Many a time, we console our friends who are grieving with statements like, 'You know what, you'll feel better soon,' or, 'You'll move on eventually.' But the issue with these statements is that these don't necessarily empower or bring comfort to a person, much less help them go through the process of grief. Our grief does not lessen with time. It is not just about moving on or 'forgetting' that makes us feel better, and it is certainly not about finding closure. After all, we never really forget the things that happen to us from the day we are born. Our muscles have memories, as does our heart.

So, how can we grieve more effectively? Firstly, we all need a safe space and time to be alone or to get the right help for ourselves to process these difficult emotions. This requires us to be present to the grief, to the loss, and to the sudden new reality that we need to adapt to and live by. Part of grieving comes with acceptance, forgiveness, and learning—accepting what is present at this very moment, the changes between the new life and the old, finding forgiveness, especially with ourselves, and learning the lessons that came with the experience so that we can truly gain closure and find completion, rather than brushing and rushing off, thinking that we have moved on. It is certainly difficult, confronting these complex feelings, and that's why we have learnt to deny them. Just because we don't think about them does not mean we don't feel them. Importantly, we have to remember that grief has no timeline, and time does not heal all wounds.

People who are grieving often end up in a cycle of self-blame, where they wish that the loss never happened. This is the stage of bargaining. When we start justifying our part in the loss, self-blame kicks in. One of the lessons of grief is to accept and to forgive. Accept that things have already happened, and that even if you could change the outcome if you did things differently, the fact of the matter is that you didn't, and the moment has already passed. We can't turn back time. Forgiving yourself comes with making peace with what has happened, realizing your place and the choices you have made or not made, and the consequences that came with it.

Forgiveness also means acknowledging that whatever you did, you did to the best of your ability as much as you could in that given moment. Every moment in our life presents lessons to learn and take away. We can never move forward with the newfound lessons in one chapter of life if we do not forgive. We may be tempted to stay and hold on to the past—but do also consider that moving forward opens new possibilities to discover a new path to walk on.

The process of dealing with grief is never just about moving on. And it is definitely not about returning things to 'normalcy', where everything looks and feels the same except for the loss and emptiness. The insistence of being in denial—trying to return things to what they were, will only make you aware of the black hole of loss and emptiness within, because the loss becomes that much more real and shocking in this fragmented reality. The process of dealing with grief is about moving forward. We move forward only by accepting things for what they are, so that we can get to where we need to go. We move forward when we don't treat our grief as our enemy. We move forward when we don't impose timelines on ourselves. We find it easier to move forward if only we allow ourselves to feel, instead of brushing our feelings aside. We move forward when we don't try to forget, reject, or suppress these difficult emotions and memories. We move forward when we allow ourselves to grieve freely, as we integrate the lessons from the experience.

When we are able to look back on what we have lost with gratitude—for the memories, for the moments we have shared, for the experience and the wisdom we have gained—we become capable of bringing the gifts we have received from grief to the next chapter of our lives, and welcome new possibilities and new beginnings.

So don't be afraid of grief. Find the space you need. Get help.

CHAPTER 1

The Complex Dynamics of the Whole Mental Health Landscape

By Dr Siew Kum Yew, Clinical Director & Clinical Psychologist, Shan You Counselling Centre

Dr Siew Kum Yew talks about the complexities in the mental health landscape—where conditions typically occur on a spectrum for people and affect their functionalities differently; how the mental health services in Singapore are heavily skewed towards a medicalized approach that does not actually help the person to change his or her core beliefs; and that our life experiences interact and reinforce one another to influence our overall mental health. Dr Siew highlights that mental health conditions do not exist in a vacuum. They occur in the context of a person's life, which involves other aspects such as work, school, relationships with family and friends, financial stress, and adverse or traumatic experiences in the past.

SEPARATING MENTAL HEALTH CONDITIONS AND THE ABILITY TO FUNCTION

MK

Can you share with me a little bit about the work that you do at Shan You Counselling Centre and what this whole centre is about?

Dr Siew

I'm the Clinical Director of Shan You Counselling Centre. At our centre, we provide counselling services to the community. Because our counselling services are partially funded by yearly grants from the Community Chest, we are able to provide the services at subsidized rates compared to, say, a private practice. The clients that we work with present a wide spectrum of issues, which include mental health issues like stress, anxiety, depression, trauma, grief and bereavement. Many of our clients present with self-harm risks, self-harm behaviour and suicide risks as well. Besides mental health issues, we also work with couples with relationship issues as well as families, mostly in terms of parenting issues.

Besides counselling services, we run a public education campaign on mental health and suicide prevention. That's our *Elephant in Our Community* public education campaign, which was launched in July 2018. The campaign aims to empower individuals and families affected by mental health conditions to seek help and live well. This year, as part of this public education campaign, we're developing *Ycare: Walking in their Shoes*, a project to increase awareness of mental health issues, suicide risks, and early warning signs of suicide among young persons. We hope that *Ycare* can help reduce the social stigma associated with mental health issues and empower young persons with mental health challenges to seek help and take better care of their mental health. We plan to launch *Ycare* on 10 September this year, in support of World Suicide Prevention Day. We hope to prevent youth suicide in the community. The truth is that every youth suicide could have been prevented. Often, they are just looking for a way out of their pain and despair but feel helpless and hopeless at the time. As a community, we can do more to prevent the next youth suicide.

MK

Got it. So, having worked with these people from all walks of life, what are some of these stigmas around mental health and suicide that you've observed on a personal level?

Dr Siew

On a personal level? Okay so, it just happened that over the course of the past two to three weeks, I've been working with five individuals who have contributed their stories and life experiences to the *Ycare* project. I'll just share a bit about some of the stigmas they have mentioned.

[Dr Siew looks up information]

Dr Siew

Okay so, one of the individuals shared that—and unfortunately, this relates to stigma at a more systemic institutional level—she has been experiencing significant mental health conditions for a number of years and was on medication. She was on the road to recovery to some extent, and she applied to a ministry for a scholarship. She went through the first round of interviews for the scholarship, and she was informed to proceed to the second phase, which included a medical review by a doctor who asked her whether she's on any medication or not. And of course, she said, 'Oh, I'm currently on medication for depression; it's an antidepressant.' And the doctor said, 'Why did you not declare that previously?' Then she said, 'Oh, there's no opportunity for me to declare it previously because nobody asked.' She mentioned the antidepressants she was on as part of the treatment she was receiving for her depression. And what happened after that was the ministry informed her that they were not going to offer her the scholarship without indicating the reason *lah*. To me, just based on the story of this individual, it seems that because of her mental health condition, she was not successful in obtaining the scholarship even though she passed phase one. So there seems to be some anxiety, some fear about giving scholarships to someone that has a history of mental health conditions. And after she declared that she was on antidepressants, there was no assessment of her mental health condition by a mental health professional to see whether she was suitable to continue with the scholarship application.

MK

It's quite problematic.

Dr Siew

It is, it is. It becomes a negative cycle because if this stigma is expressed at both the community level and the institutional level, then it's very natural for people with mental health conditions to not tell people about it. And so, if people know that they will be disadvantaged when they tell a prospective employer or someone in authority that they have a mental health condition, then they will not say, right? And if they do not say, then it is less likely that they'll get the support that they need when they're working in that organization. It's less likely that they will be . . .

MK

. . . Supported in an environment where they can heal or even reconcile with themselves.

Dr Siew

Yes, I think in this sense, we need to separate the person's ability to function, do their work, or study, from their mental health condition. If we really want to be inclusive then we need to be open to talking about mental health conditions and how, if you declare a mental health condition, an organization or place can support you.

MK

Instead of saying 'you're not suited for this role' even if the person has proven to have the abilities to do so. I don't know where to start. And even looking for support is hard when you know that you're in deep waters, because there are certain notions that you can't share with people, in order to protect yourself and the people around you.

Dr Siew

And it's rational. So that's one of the reasons, if you actually look at the Singapore Mental Health Study in 2016,[2] it found that more than three-quarters of people with mental health issues do not seek professional help. That's the treatment gap in our community.

But then there is also another important issue about treatment delay. So, in terms of treatment delay for a person that has Major Depressive Disorder, based on the Singapore Mental Health Study

---

[2] M. Subramaniam, E. Abdin, J. A. Vaingankar, S. Shafie, B.Y. Chua, R. Sambasivam, Y. J. Zhang, et al., 'Tracking the Mental Health of a Nation: Prevalence and Correlates of Mental Disorders in the Second Singapore Mental Health Study', *Epidemiology and Psychiatric Sciences* 29, 2020: e29. doi:10.1017/S2045796019000179.

2016, the delay is about a year between the onset of depressive symptoms and seeking treatment. Bipolar Disorder is four years. For Generalized Anxiety Disorder, it's about two years. And treatment delay for alcohol abuse is four years. So, stigma also contributes to treatment delay. And of course, we know that if you are stuck experiencing mental health issues that are impairing your day-to-day functioning, the earlier you seek support or effective professional help from psychiatrists, psychologists, counsellors, or art therapists, the higher the likelihood that you can actually recover fully and faster from those mental health struggles.

MK

Got it. What are some of the other stories that you have?

Dr Siew

I just want to highlight an experience of social stigma associated with suicide that is not really talked about often. This is a story of a mother who lost her only child to suicide. When it happened, she experienced quite explicit stigmatizing responses from her family, her relatives, and her neighbours. The neighbours looked at her differently, avoided talking to her, and her relatives did not even want to talk about the death of her son.

This mother also experienced some sort of self-stigma. Social stigma is the discriminating attitudes and beliefs that people in a society have towards something. Self-stigma happens when a person internalizes these discriminating attitudes and believes them to be true about themselves and, as a result, feels ashamed. When there is a strong social stigma associated with mental health issues and suicide in the community, and when it happens to your own child, the social stigma that you learnt from society becomes internalized as your self-stigma. So, the mother was having a really difficult time after she lost her only child to suicide. Not only was there immense grief from losing her child, but there was also the self-stigma and shame from losing a child to suicide. There were many weeks and months of thinking, 'Was I a bad mother? Could I have done something differently? What did I do wrong?' The mother experienced a lot of guilt and shame coming from within herself and from the people around her.

MK

A lot of bereaved mums have experienced the same things as well.

Dr Siew

Yes. When you're a bereaved mum and you've lost a child to suicide, you're not just dealing with the usual grief and bereavement.

MK

You're also dealing with the societal frameworks around it.

Dr Siew

You're dealing with the social stigma, and the self-stigma associated with losing a child to suicide.

THE ACTUAL COST OF MENTAL HEALTH ISSUES

MK

What is really holding people back from seeking help or support? It's a chicken and egg question . . . But based on your experience and all these different stories that you've accumulated, what are some of the interventions that you think we can consider implementing so that we can reduce these stigmas? So that we can bring together people who are really in need of support? So that the resources that are available can be distributed?

Dr Siew

I think society, organizations and companies need to understand, at a broader level, the cost associated with someone with a mental health condition.

At a societal level, if someone is experiencing mental health difficulties and does not receive appropriate, effective help to cope and recover from the condition, and continues to experience it for a long period of time, for years, for decades, then society as a whole needs to look at what the cost is. What's the economic loss to society? The loss of employment to society, the loss of work productivity. And there's the social cost as well, because if a member of society has a mental health condition, the person with the mental health condition will also impact the family and the quality of relationship with other members of the family. And of course, if you want to go further, if the person doesn't recover from the condition, he or she is less likely to get into a relationship and form a family. So, these are very clear and long-term costs to the community.

At the organizational level, if you have an employee with a mental health issue, and he or she doesn't talk about it or the company doesn't help the person and support in his or her recovery, and if the issue is exacerbated by stress, there is loss in terms of what the person can contribute to the company. If we understand this cost, then the funding that needs to be channelled to help someone recover from mental health conditions actually becomes a small percentage of the company's total operating cost.

Mental health issues are not always serious mental health conditions like schizophrenia or depression. If you help people cope better with their mental health, then everybody benefits! Let's say a young person dies by suicide at the age of twenty. That, of course, is tragic and sad for the young person and his or her family and friends. But there is also a real economic cost associated with that loss. If on average he earns $60k a year, over ten years, we're talking about earnings of $600k. Over twenty years, it's $1.2 million. So that's the real economic loss to the family and to society. It's about whether society, the government and companies can see this bigger picture and start taking mental health issues seriously, and support their people and employees and staff with mental health issues more rigorously.

And organizations can do more. They can look at how to reduce institutional stigma. This stigma is about the policies of organizations that discriminate against persons with mental health issues. Such institutional stigma is common across all types of organizations, and sadly, including those that provide mental health services. Many people with mental health conditions face significant barriers when seeking employment. Employees are often concerned about being discriminated against at work and therefore don't seek professional help.

THE GAP THAT MEDICATION DOESN'T RESOLVE

MK

Is there anything else you want to speak out on regarding the current situation we're dealing with? Be it mental health, or suicide prevention.

Dr Siew

What has been said by quite a few people in the past—and one of the people who has said that is Anthea Ong—is that the mental health services in Singapore are heavily skewed towards a medicalized approach. And that is an approach that has a historical context in Singapore. The issue with an overly medicalized approach is that when a psychiatrist prescribes medications to someone with a mental health condition, the medication actually does not help the person to change his or her thinking, his or her core belief, how the person responds to mental health symptoms or stresses in the environment, or how the person deals with past traumatic memories.

There are mental health conditions that have a strong neurophysiological basis. When there's a neurophysiological imbalance causing a mental health condition, medication is very important in addressing this imbalance. Psychiatric medications work on the neurotransmitters in the brain that regulate our mood and thinking. Research has shown that neurophysiological imbalances in the brain contribute to mental health conditions such as schizophrenia and bipolar disorder. For these conditions, medication is very important. But even for persons with schizophrenia and bipolar disorder, psychotherapy and counselling are also very important in helping the person respond well to the distress and difficulties that he or she may be experiencing so that they can focus on long-term recovery through changes in behaviour and choices.

For some conditions, medication can improve clinical symptoms so that counselling is more effective. To illustrate, medication could help to improve some symptoms of clinical depression, such as insomnia, fatigue, and difficulty in paying attention, thereby helping the person to respond better in counselling.

However, the key factor in mental health recovery is really about how the person responds to what is happening in the mind and the external environment—whatever thoughts that are triggered, whatever core beliefs one may have, whatever emotions one may be experiencing. Medication does not help someone alter their thinking, perspectives and beliefs about who they are, and how they relate to other people and the world.

And if someone has a mental health condition that has a stronger psychological and emotional basis, then counselling and psychotherapy would be more important in helping the person understand and unpack what is happening in the mind and in his or her life, and to see how to respond in a way that is helpful and would facilitate recovery.

MK

Got it, got it. What was very powerful was how you made the distinctions very clearly in terms of which methodology to use. Because these days, one of the things is there's a lot of misinformation out there. For example, people read three articles about depression and mental health and start diagnosing themselves—even if they may just be dealing with their own stress, for example. There needs to be more precise *judgement* of where we are at, so that we know which methodology will actually apply to us and effectively create the necessary healing.

Dr Siew

Yes. There's another mental health condition, social anxiety disorder, that causes extreme anxiety and fear in social settings. People with this condition may have difficulty meeting new people and attending work meetings or social gatherings. They fear being judged or assessed by other people. But anxiety in social settings is also something that we all experience to some degree. When you're meeting someone for the first time, you may experience anxiety about how you look or how the other person may be judging you in some way. Very often, our experiences of anxiety are linked to what we have learnt from previous experiences. For example, if your father had criticized you for not doing well in school in the past, when you attend a job interview as an adult, certain negative automatic thoughts learnt from that past experience can be triggered during the interview . . .

MK

And you start projecting even against your best judgement. You can't help but feel those emotions that are present, just like how they were, once upon a time, when your dad made those remarks.

Dr Siew

Yes, correct. But there are different levels of social anxiety. In the context of a job interview, we all experience some anxiety, but if the anxiety is not really affecting our ability to do well in the interview, then that is fine—such anxiety is normal. But for some people, because the social anxiety has developed over many years and across many adverse and anxiety-provoking experiences, it has developed to an extent that the social anxiety affects the person's ability to do well in a job interview. The person may start to have rapid heart palpitations, may start to tremble, may blush and sweat excessively, and may have difficulty thinking and speaking clearly during the interview. Social anxiety impairs the person's functioning. If you give medication to this person, it will not help them understand and unpack why they are experiencing this excessive anxiety. What are the negative automatic thoughts that are triggered? What are the underlying core beliefs that have developed over the years from past adverse experiences? How should they respond to those unhelpful thoughts and beliefs? When one's thinking, core beliefs, and responses change, one can progressively recover from the social anxiety disorder. But medication doesn't do that.

MK

Why?

Dr Siew

Because medication only works on the neurophysiological system of the brain and body and that's just the physical body. But what . . .

MK

. . . What we're dealing with are the mental and emotional bodies.

Dr Siew

Yes—medication works on the neurobiological system of the body, the physiology of the body. But what is more complex than the physical body is the mind, the consciousness. The mind is very complex. The mind contains many experiences and mental phenomena that we commonly come to understand as thoughts, emotions, bodily sensations, memories, urges, and impulses. And all these are experienced in the mind, and there are a lot of these things happening in the mind from moment to moment to moment. If we want to help someone with mental health challenges that are basically experienced in the mind, we would need more than medication.

WHAT LIES BEHIND THE CRIME?

MK

Tell me a little bit more about the work that you do with the people in prison. Part of talking about stigmas is also recognizing that some of these people are considered outcasts by the general population because of the things they did in the past. How are they recovering? What are some of the stigmas that are still present? I'm asking more about the psychology behind that, because mental health involves that as well.

Dr Siew

There are actually a few aspects to understand. One is the forensic aspect, the criminal aspect. For example, I go into a shop and steal a handphone because I want to have a newer, better handphone, or I want to sell the handphone in order to get some money to, let's say, buy a branded sports shoe. That is because of greed or desire, and that is clearly due to forensic issues, criminal issues.

But the life of someone who committed a criminal offence is much more complex than that. Very often, what you'll find is that a lot of them have had adverse early life experiences. Common things they've experienced are psychological abuse, emotional abuse, physical abuse, or sexual abuse at the hands of adults in their family or social settings. And as a result, they develop mental health issues that subsequently contribute to them not doing well in life. And because they don't do well in life, they have been sidelined by society, they go down a difficult path, and tend to gravitate towards social groups that have a more negative influence on them. And they get a sense of belonging and sense of self-esteem from these social groups.

But what is often not highlighted are the mental health issues that contribute to people committing criminal offences. In the example of stealing a handphone, the person may go into a shop to steal a handphone because the act of stealing may provide some form of psychological or emotional relief to the person. The person may feel better in some way after stealing the handphone, even if he or she doesn't need it. What triggers the stealing behaviour is the need to have a sense of accomplishment because the person who is stealing is maybe very stressed, or very down. The act of stealing helps to provide some temporary psychological and emotional relief from the low mood. Another pathway is when the mental health condition, like clinical depression, diminishes the ability of the individual to manage certain negative impulses or think about the consequences of his or her behaviour.

These issues are complex, and they often interact with and reinforce one another. Experiencing adverse life events, especially during childhood, and mental health issues often increase the risks of offending behaviours later in life. Breaking the vicious cycle is often tough for someone with an entrenched mix of adverse childhood events, mental health issues, family conflicts, and multiple incarcerations. We need to know the person's life story in order to begin to understand his or her behaviour.

LISTEN, RELATE, EMPATHIZE

MK

If we look at it as a whole, it's still a vicious cycle. I'm wondering, what do you think we can do as a collective? Because one person doing something is not enough. We have to rally people from all walks of life to come together to play a part in this.

If someone is experiencing or living with a mental health condition or with some significant mental health challenges, what everyone should understand is that there are very complex dynamics involved. Mental health conditions do not exist in a vacuum. They occur in the context of a person's life, which involves aspects like work, school, relationships with the family, with friends, financial stress, whether the person suffered adverse or traumatic experiences in the past, and all that.

Dr Siew

Mental health conditions do not just appear overnight. They typically evolve over a period of time, from months to years, during which the person would likely have experienced multiple adverse or traumatic events. There are very complex dynamics at play, and it's very difficult for people to understand all the complexities. The simple answer to your question is that it's important for all of us to learn to connect well with each other, to really listen, to talk to someone without judging—because we have not lived that person's life. We have not walked a day in that person's shoes. We have not had that person's experience, so we can't judge whether that person is good or bad, or weak or strong.

MK

We cannot look at it from a morality space.

Dr Siew

Yes, and we cannot look at it as whether the person is weak or failing to cope with the challenges of life, because we have not lived the person's life. What had led to that point or that moment in the person's life? What had led to that experience on that particular day?

In our mind, we often judge our experiences and other people automatically, because our judging thoughts and judging beliefs are triggered automatically. This is normal. This is just the nature of the mind, as our thoughts and beliefs about life and people have been conditioned from our past experiences since childhood. When we become aware that we are judging, we should try to just hold it in our awareness and not express it in our interactions and relationships with someone. The first step is to be present, and to listen and connect without judging. If we can do that, we can then relate to the person with empathy, with kindness, and with compassion.

And it will actually help, if we do so as a collective, to break invisible vicious cycles in our community. Whether it's a vicious cycle associated with someone who has committed a criminal offence, or someone who is experiencing mental health challenges. As a collective, if we're able to do that, and as a country, if we're able to direct more resources and funding to help people with mental health challenges, to help people who have committed criminal offences—then as a collective, we can break these cycles together. It's about supporting people and uplifting them to a positive path in life, one that gives hope for a better future. Breaking these invisible vicious cycles in the community requires us to form integrated and empowering solutions across our mental health services, social service agencies, the education system, the criminal justice system, as well as governmental institutions, so that we can adequately respond to the challenges that people face in their daily lives.

In our daily lives, let's try to be more understanding that many people are experiencing challenges that we don't know of. Let's try to be more understanding if there are delays, or if things don't go smoothly at work. We can be kinder, more patient with others, and look out for each other's wellbeing. I think we need to ask ourselves, what kind of society do we want our children and their children to live in? And what are we doing about it now?

THE SECRET TO PREVENTING BURNOUT

Dr Siew

When I'm talking to my team of psychologists and counsellors about what is important to progress in the helping profession, it is the ability to relate to your clients or your patients in a way that is authentic, real, and genuine. When you're in sessions with your client, be present. Someone once said to me, 'The most important thing that you can give a person is your full attention and be present to the person.' And that is fundamental to the work of a psychologist or a counsellor. If you want to be effective in helping a person, you need to be present and respond in an empathetic way to the person you are talking to and helping.

And the other important value is to have a sense of the purpose of the work. And that sense of purpose of the work can be defined quite simply: *In this session, in this moment, what can I say, or what can I do that can best help this client or this patient with his or her difficulties or distress?* That is the sense of purpose of the work in that moment. On a broader level, the purpose of the work is, to define it simply, to alleviate the pain, suffering, and distress of your clients, and to help facilitate positive change and growth in them.

And another important part of the work is to develop certain clinical competencies and skills that work. If you want to help someone with anxiety disorders, with depression, with bipolar disorder, you need to have adequate clinical competencies and skills in therapeutic interventions that have been shown to be effective in research studies, as well as the ability to deliver these therapeutic interventions in a way that works for the client sitting in front of you. And once you have some level of mastery of the competencies, skills and abilities needed to be effective in helping, you will then have the recurrent experience of a sense of fulfilment, a sense of satisfaction, and a sense that there's meaning and purpose in your work. And that sense of fulfilment, meaning and purpose and satisfaction in your work is actually the best protection against burnout.

MK

Yes!

Dr Siew

So, you're genuine, you're authentic, you're present, you come from this sense of purpose, and you don't allow whatever dysfunctional ego that you have to impact how you relate to your client in that moment, because it is not about you! It's about what can best benefit this client in front of you, in this moment, in this session.

And that's not easy because it takes a journey of many years to develop the competencies and skills through attending trainings, self-reflection, case discussions, supervision, and all that. Once you have some level of mastery in the necessary competencies and skills, the ability to be authentic and present and respond with empathy to the person in front of you, not only will you find a recurrent sense of fulfilment, satisfaction, joy, and meaning in your work, but also any mental health or helping service will want you.

I think people who want to become a helping professional or a mental health professional need to understand that having good intentions is not good enough to be an effective and competent helper who can do the work for many years. All that I mentioned is important and often not emphasized enough when the person undergoes postgraduate training in counselling or psychology. Because the postgraduate training tends to be more focused on theory and on the academic and research aspect. There is not enough emphasis on developing all these important values that are needed to become a competent and effective helper.

The counsellors and psychologists in training are not really valued for their ability to relate and connect with others in an authentic and deep way. But I do understand why, in most postgraduate trainings in counselling or psychology, theoretical and research knowledge and technical competency are emphasized. While these domains are also important in any postgraduate training, they are more easily assessed in terms of whether a student meets a satisfactory level of competency and knowledge in the subject matter. I think what's important is that helping organizations support professionals develop all these aspects that I mentioned earlier.

Once there is less concern about whether your career or job is affected by your professional opinion or your professional position in certain subject matters, more mental health professionals would be willing to express their real professional opinions and perspectives about important areas in our mental health landscape. Then, together, as a collective of mental health professionals, psychologists, counsellors, social workers, case managers, or psychiatrists, we can collectively voice our diverse opinions or perspectives in a way that would bring about real changes to the community, and to governmental and institutional policies.

CHAPTER 2

Creating Safe Spaces to Honour Our Mental Health as a Nation

By Brenda Lee and Lynn Tan, Clinical Psychologists, The Psychology Practice

Is therapy only for the broken and privileged? The conversation opened with a reflection by Brenda Lee and Lynn Tan on the reasons people do not seek help. Some people feel that going to therapy means that something is wrong with them, which is a barrier that hinders them from being open to the idea. Others might also view therapy as a service only for the privileged. Mental health education needs to start young in order to dispel these myths. Ultimately, Brenda and Lynn stress the importance of creating safe spaces not only in the therapy room but in the community at large, so that people can express their emotions and develop a better awareness of mental and emotional health.

IS THERAPY ONLY FOR THE BROKEN AND PRIVILEGED?

MK

What do you think is really holding people back from seeking help?

Brenda

I think part of it is mental health literacy. Even though in recent times more has been done, you do still see the gaps today where people do not know where to seek help, or don't quite understand or have a clear idea of what it is they're experiencing. Sometimes you have people coming in and they'll say, 'Oh yeah I haven't really thought about seeking help because I thought it's just something that would go away on its own or it's something that isn't a problem, that it's just the way things are.' One of the things then, is having more awareness of mental wellness, what it entails, and the resources and avenues that are available.

I think there's also this idea—and this is probably more prominent when working in the public hospital setting—where there's a lot of, *if I come here, if I see you, it must mean I'm crazy, there's something wrong with me.* I suppose more people cognitively know that it's not the case, but the emotional attachment to the idea of *there must be something wrong* or *I'm crazy* seems to still be sticking in some ways, if that makes sense.

MK

It does.

Lynn

And on the other side of the coin, there's also a population who feels that receiving therapy is a luxury only for the privileged. We do get different ends of the spectrum in terms of what they associate therapy or seeking help with. But building on, what Brenda also said, mental health and emotional literacy is something we could do a lot more of in our upbringing and education system. Where do we learn how to label these experiences we are experiencing in our bodies? Can we normalize them? And perhaps learn to consider what emotional needs are unmet? The reality for most of us growing up is that this isn't something that has been adequately nurtured and cultivated, so it becomes *oh I'm experiencing this thing, I don't have any words or vocabulary to describe this experience* and then it becomes *since I don't know, I push it away*, or *I will not use it as information to attend to what exactly I need in the moment.*

START EXPLORING EMOTIONAL LITERACY TODAY

MK

I'm just wondering, what are some interventions on a community level within our ecosystem that we can do more of, to participate at a higher level? Be it in the public or private sector.

Brenda

The first thing that came to mind was what Lynn mentioned earlier about emotional literacy. While a fair amount has been done in recent years to dispel myths and raise awareness about mental health, including different conditions such as depression, OCD[3], etc., a lot more can be done in terms of looking at how we can start building mastery of our emotions and cultivate emotional literacy from a young age. This can be incorporated into the school curriculum in some ways. And also, educating and equipping parents with the tools to do so. I feel this would be something worthwhile and meaningful to look into.

[3] OCD: Obsessive Compulsive Disorder

Lynn

I think to add to what Brenda said, while it is important to start young, we can certainly also start from where people are at. Take leaders leading in our present climate, for example. COVID-19 is accompanied by a lot of disconnection—emotional disconnection, physical disconnection, social disconnection. It is so important to be emotionally attuned to your own needs, but for leaders, it is also about being attuned to the people who are supporting them and people they're working with. As leaders, when we are not attuned to what is happening on the ground and across levels in the organization, it's easy to overlook symptoms of burnout. Jennifer Moss wrote an article[4] for the *Harvard Business Review* in February this year exploring COVID-19 and burnout. They surveyed 1,500 respondents across forty-six countries in various industries and seniority levels. It revealed that burnout was experienced globally, with respondents reporting deteriorating wellbeing and work-life balance, and increasing job demands and workload. She emphasized changing organizational practices and culture to balance out the present individual bottom-up initiatives such as mindfulness and yoga. We need to consider issues with a sharper intersectional lens to better identify populations who are more vulnerable in a crisis. If we start emotional literacy training or exploration now, where people are at, we'll probably find ourselves in a better place to attend to our own needs and a better place to be sensitive to the needs of others.

HOW CAN WE LISTEN TO DIFFERENT VOICES IN SOCIETY?

Lynn

But to address Ming Kwang's original question on what can be done other than emotional literacy, I think the other thing that's

---

[4] Jennifer Moss, 'Beyond Burned Out', *Harvard Business Review*, 2021, https://hbr.org/2021/02/beyond-burned-out.

coming up and keeps sticking in my head is being more accepting of voices of dissent and diversity. When I think about mental health stigma, it brings to mind an association with intolerance towards diversity. For example, neuro-diversity, able-ness, cultural diversity, etc. Have our systems been encouraging towards different voices, or have we been leaning towards homogeneity? In February this year, there was an article published in *Current Biology* describing parachute science in marine science research.[5] The authors spoke of a practice of scientists from higher-income countries 'parachuting' into lower-income countries to conduct research and eventually publishing it, without adequate engagement with native researchers. This practice may not only hamper local research efforts but also create dependency on external expertise. Furthermore, research questions may fail to sensitively address local needs. How did this occur? Lack of funding? Has our published scientific literature better served one population over another? It really gets me thinking about what sort of data we are missing out on. Circling back to psychology, much of our normative data for our psychological tools is from research conducted in the West. The question stands: whose voices are left behind in society, policy, academia, and in the services that we offer? Can we move deliberately to amplify diverse voices?

Brenda

Along these lines, do we have the space, or can we look into having spaces where we can have voices of dissent and diversity? But I think we need to also think about where our society is at and how receptive they would be to something like this. Diversity can be viewed as something that would go against a lot of what has been inculcated in us, given the uniqueness of Singapore's circumstances. Now, we're almost talking about the national

[5] Paris V. Stefanoudis et al., 'Turning the tide of parachute science', *Current Biology* 31, no. 4 (2021): R184–R185, https://doi.org/10.1016/j.cub.2021.01.029.

level: the common narrative that we've always been told is that we're a small nation, we can't afford to have too many voices of dissent. And the very fact that right now I'm saying this, and how much hesitation I'm experiencing saying this, is probably saying a lot as well, if it makes sense.

MK

Yeah, it does.

Brenda

So definitely what Lynn is saying makes a lot of sense, and it's what we need to work towards but at the same time, it is a tricky process that requires people to come together. Like what we're doing right now, you inviting us, being able to talk about it is one of those tiny steps towards that direction but definitely, more people need to come together on different levels. I think we need to think about how this can be done in a way that wouldn't shut people down or threaten people's sense of security while facilitating much needed acceptance of diversity and differing views.

Lynn

I think it's partly what's drawn us to your initiative, Ming Kwang. I think the initiative that you have started is encouraging a lot of diverse voices coming together as a community to create a little jigsaw puzzle of what we need as a society to start questioning and asking, *Hey, are certain systems serving us well?* And while I understand where Brenda is coming from—I sense that it's big and scary—it is these small steps that make a difference. It's really asking, *Hey, why are we doing certain things a certain way and merely following along just because it's the norm?*

It's asking ourselves, *Hey just because it's the norm, does it mean that it's right?* Are we also subtly silencing certain voices, or are we only allowing certain individuals to come in because they are privileged or they have the means to come in? Even in a space like

psychology for example, it's predominantly female. Is our space not safe enough for our male counterparts to join us? I'm just thinking out loud. What voices are we leaving behind, and are there small little things that we can do to start shifting or questioning the status quo? It doesn't have to be big. It doesn't have to be at the policy level, although policies would help. I think if we were to start thinking about our decision-making more intentionally and questioning the status quo, that would encourage more diversity.

SAFETY AS A PREREQUISITE FOR VULNERABILITY

MK

It makes a lot of sense. We talked a lot about community and national interventions. Let's bring it down to the individual level. What can individuals do to better manage their mental and emotional wellness?

Brenda

I think the idea of staying in touch with your emotions is coming up more often these days, or it's an emerging theme. Being able to have that awareness of *what am I feeling and why may I be feeling the way I am*. Having the language to describe it, label it, communicate or express it as well, and being able to then listen in to what our emotions are telling us. For instance, when I'm feeling sad, how am I experiencing it in my body? What is this sadness I'm feeling, telling me about what I need? This is something that I feel is applicable to anyone. You don't need to have emotional difficulties or be feeling unwell for this to be relevant.

Lynn

I guess to expand on what Brenda shared, if it's hard to access the words to describe the experience, maybe notice where in the body it resides. *I'm feeling something now, I don't have the words to describe it, that's fine, that's okay. Where in the body does it feel most saturated?* Maybe then, the words may come to me to describe the experience. Or maybe, it is easier to describe the feeling using movement, or music, or art. There are so many different ways to describe feelings aside from verbal means. I find that often in our quest to cognitively make sense of our emotions, we forget about how it impacts our bodies. When we are able to integrate information from our head, heart, and body, perhaps we can consider our emotions as merely messengers. What's anger telling me? Is it telling me that an injustice has been done? What is disappointment telling me? An unmet expectation? Asking ourselves this and being curious about our experiences—bodily experiences, emotional experiences.

[contemplative silence]

Lynn

But I think on that note, on the topic of emotions and vulnerability, we also ought to talk about safety because that cannot happen without feeling safe. If we don't feel safe in our bodies, if we do not feel safe in the spaces or the people we connect with, how can we expect ourselves to be vulnerable? I guess, when we talk about connecting to somebody, it's thinking about: *How do I listen attentively? How do I listen to understand instead of respond? How do I hold myself back in that sense and really be curious about the experience that this person is trying to tell me and convey to me? How do I create a space safe enough for this person to share?* I think that is something that is easy to say but quite hard to do. I'm finding it quite hard to put it into words because it's not as simple as saying that *this space is safe*. How do I build that trust with this individual? And it's so unique to different people. How do I build that trust, so this person feels safe enough with me to share what they're struggling with?

Brenda

That's probably something we can do for one another on an individual level. How can we contribute or create more safe spaces in the community at large other than the therapy space itself?

Lynn

How do we learn to be comfortable with sitting with big emotions? If you come back to a parent and child dynamic, when a child is crying or throwing a tantrum, how can I, as a parent, sit with my child, and be with them? It's the *being with* experience, to *be with* my child as they are learning to regulate their own feelings while trying not to intervene and change their experience. It's starting that young. How do I communicate that anger is normal, that it doesn't need to be changed? How do I suspend my own past experiences with anger and sit with you through your experience?

BRIDGING THE DEMAND AND SUPPLY GAP IN MENTAL HEALTH SERVICES

MK

There are certain limitations that people experience when seeking mental health treatments in the public sector. I feel that it is necessary to unpack this whole conversation because it is also one of the factors that stop people from getting the help they need in time before their conditions start getting worse. I'm just wondering, what are the gaps in the existing treatments in the public sector that are still left unsaid, that require more unpacking, more awareness, and more interventions? How can the private sector—whatever you guys are doing—fill in the gaps?

Lynn

I think the biggest thing that comes to mind is the wait time.

MK

Tell me more!

[Brenda laughs]

Brenda

When I was in public health, what I saw around me and what I experienced myself is that in reality, resources are finite, and oftentimes that translates into a long wait time. So let us say, you do have individuals that are seeking help, but there's always that struggle of being able to provide help or for them to receive timely help or interventions or essentially even appointments. It can be frustrating, because you want to help, but it feels almost like your hands are tied because there's only so much you can do.

Lynn

I share the same frustration as Brenda. In public health, when we were there, it's . . . ugh.

[Lynn sighs heavily]

Lynn

Even if, personally, we have the resources to reach out to help, the logistical resources are finite. There's only that many rooms available. There are only that many time slots available and I think it's *extremely* frustrating when we are, I guess, many layers down. But beyond that, I think the question you're also asking is beyond finite logistical resources, we also hold finite emotional resources. It circles back to the huge topic on burnout. There are only that many people that we can see in a day, in a week, in a month. Only that many people we can hold in our minds. We have to consider what is sustainable and ethical, so that we can effectively serve the clients that we see. Generally, however, in public health, there's this sense of lack of agency and associated feelings of frustration and helplessness: it often feels that there are too many factors that are outside of our control.

Brenda

It's a systemic issue.

MK

Is it also because there are not enough psychologists, psychotherapists, and therapists in the market from a supply and demand perspective?

Lynn

I think there is a growing demand!

Brenda

The other part you asked about is the private sector. Is that something you're still curious about?

MK

I am!

Brenda

Okay. I think in the most general sense, it's really about how we can work and communicate better with one another. Sometimes it feels almost like there's a wide gap between public and private practice. And I think that even just within our profession itself—Lynn, I don't know how you feel about this—it's something that can be bridged more. And I think this is where policies can come into play, such that there are more options available to people. So, for example, if I'm not feeling good, I'm struggling, my choices don't have to be as black and white. Currently, if my condition is really serious or if I have limited finances, it seems that my only option would be to go to a tertiary hospital. How can we look into our existing policies, and how can we invest in the mental health industry, such that the choice can be less dichotomous or less either-or, so that even if my condition is serious and/or I have limited finances, I have the option of seeing someone in private without worrying about cost or whether I would get the care and expertise that I need? I think if we are able to do that, then that can potentially lessen the load that's on the public healthcare system. At least in mental health.

Lynn

I resonate with what Brenda said. I think very often it just feels very divided. How do we bridge the gap and offer more reasonable and realistic options for clients to choose from that are well-matched to their needs? It shouldn't be at the expense of the client's time, health, finance, or choice of treatment.

LEARNING HOW TO CREATE SAFE SPACES

MK

Got it. Any final message to the public? What would you say to the public if you have a message regarding mental health, emotional wellness, and suicide prevention you wish to spread and inculcate out there?

[Brenda laughs]

Brenda

That's a big question!

[silence]

Lynn

I think I keep coming back to this idea of safe spaces. How do we create safe spaces for each other and ourselves? How do we encourage, even in this, just the recent question, you're asking how we can get more diverse access, right? How do we bridge the private and public sectors? How do we encourage more diversity in the way that we practise and the way that we relate to each other? I keep coming back to this. How do we create safe spaces? And how do we build a self-reflective practice for ourselves? How do we cultivate this internal muscle to make decisions that are more sensitive and intentional, for our mental wellbeing, for our relationships and, for the wider community to have more honest and vulnerable connections?

MK

Got it. I think building safe spaces should be training that individuals have to learn. Because, to be honest, all these things about emotional literacy, creating safe spaces, even listening—we're not really trained for it. I learnt to listen only when I was getting trained as a coach. That's how I picked it up, and I realized that there are different layers to it that we are not taught. For example, it's possible to hear the unsaid, hear the emotions, hear the things that the person is not saying aloud. There are masks underneath the layers of words, and I feel that we are missing all these little trainings. I don't know whether to say the gap lies in schools, but as a curriculum, as a training, we live our lives without really knowing how to do all this. Even when we're with the other person, we're not really fully present. Most of the time we're in our heads, too quick to make judgements, too quick to make a conclusion out of things rather than be present with the other person in the space itself. And I think the first step to creating safe spaces is really about being able to be present and be there for the other person. It's like being able to hold space for the other person so that they are able to express what they have to express, whatever that means, in whatever form that takes.

Brenda

For me, it's also about how we can come together more. It's related to creating safe spaces, but it's also the idea of how we can come and work together better towards this idea of honouring our mental health as a nation. Along these lines, even when I was in public health, there were a lot of initiatives on exactly this. While there are a fair number of initiatives going on, it seems like everyone is working in silos and that puzzled me so much because I'm thinking, why can't we then come together so that there is less overlapping and increased ability to harness what we can collectively bring to the table?

Lynn

I think what happens is it's like a competition of who has the best initiative. Then the cause, the spirit, the heart of it gets lost. I think it's asking ourselves: instead of competing with each other, how can we lift each other up? How can we support each other better? Because when we start to compete, we lose voices. How can we lift each other up and move away from competition and towards collaboration? I remember we had many conversations about that.

MK

Got it. Thank you so much, I hope you found this valuable. It was very interesting.

CHAPTER 3

Enabling Mental Health and Wellbeing across All Career Stages

By Patrick Tay, Member of Parliament, Chairperson of Pioneer SMC

Patrick Tay shares the various ways mental health stigmas occur in the workplace from three groups: entry into employment, those already in employment, and those leaving employment. Each group faces its own set of stressors and stigmas, and we have to consider the kind of support each needs. He highlights that fundamentally, we must avoid discriminatory practices, and that HR and employers need to be more aware of their employee's mental wellbeing and regulate arrangements, especially so during COVID-19.

A LAYERED AND INTERCONNECTED ISSUE

Patrick

At a local level, being a Member of Parliament and looking after constituencies from Yishun, Boon Lay, and Pioneer SMC particularly this past year after COVID, I do see more issues of fatigue showing up. Mental health covers a very broad spectrum, so mental fatigue could lead to mental health issues. On various fronts: it could be neighbourly disputes due to stress, job losses, or even issues in the family. In particular, mental fatigue has increased as we work from home. And as a matter of fact, not everybody has the luxury of owning a big home with few people. Some people live with their extended family. Some people live with their tenants. Some people live with their parents, or their grandparents, or even with three generations. And that can turn out to be quite exacting. Today, as we're having this conversation, it has just been announced that we are opening up to 75 per cent of the workplace on Monday (7 April 2021). Yet, still, in the new normal, I feel that mental fatigue is something we need to be watchful and mindful of, especially on a community level.

Coming from the NTUC Labor Movement, mental health issues are very important in the workplace for a variety of reasons at various levels. It could be, for example, when hiring a selection of people with mental health conditions, whether they will be discriminated against, or how receptive employers are to people with pre-existing mental health conditions.

Another one is about fatigue and excessive stress, especially now when we work from home and have back-to-back meetings. Some people who work globally have complained to me: 'Daytime nine to five I'm with my local boss, but because I'm connected to the US, at 7.00 pm, I have to go online again because everyone wants to do the Zoom at their local time'. So, we have various challenges, and us being globalized only exacerbates things. I think the other one is mental health issues because of work. Singapore is stressful enough with various exacting demands: family, commitments, work, and all the lines between work and family become blurred because of work from home restrictions. So that creates a certain level of mental health issues at the workplace.

Mental health is a focus for the Ministry of Manpower and Tripartite Partners. It is classified under the umbrella of workplace safety and health. We recently came up with a Tripartite Alliance, and we are cognizant of the fact that because of work from home arrangements, it may spin off into other bigger challenges. Thus, we're trying to plug the gap there.

And finally for the last part, recruitment selection—and that includes hiring and re-employment, how that affects mental health, and how it may be quite traumatic for people who are terminated and retrenched. I've been involved in many retrenchments in the last nineteen years, from SARS to the global financial crisis to now COVID-19. Sometimes it's our Asian culture that is a bit less forgiving when people go through these tough times. It's an esteem issue, and it may border to depressive behaviours and negative thought patterns. So, these are the various fronts.

If I may say, I think mental health is something that is multi-ministerial, and the MOH[6] is driving it very intensely. When I was in the GPC[7] for Health, I was always pushing the ante in this area, and it stretches across ministries. The Ministry of Health, of course, is in partnership with the Ministry of Manpower because of the workplace, and that also feeds into the Ministry of Social and Family Development because it's in a local community. Mental health is now—

[6] MOH: Ministry of Health

[7] GPC: Government Parliamentary Committee

MK

It's more dynamic now, it's no longer just about health.

Patrick

And now, there's a fourth one—the Ministry of Education! As I'm in the GPC for Education, I recently just spoke about it during the latest Committee of Supply Debate for the GPC for Education, where I gave five big points and ideas. I spoke on mental health and wellness at schools. Now, the MOE[8] looks over everything from kindergarten to continuous education and training. So how can we overcome this? We hear of so many suicide cases. I'm concerned. There's bullying, there's suicides, or attempted suicides, and of course, a number of patients that are seeking treatment. We have IMH[9], and I'm quite familiar with the mental health treatment facility there because I used to be the Executive Secretary of Healthcare Services Employees' Union, so I did interact with the people at IMH quite frequently, and I'm totally aware of its effects on people. Young people have their own set of issues. The older ones also have issues because of dementia, and therefore, the term 'mental health' covers a big spectrum. I didn't realize it's so broad. I'm not a doctor by training, but if you really classify it, there's quite a long list of conditions that border around mental health illnesses.

MK

And then these days we have a new problem—people self-diagnosing themselves.

Patrick

You see that?

[8] MOE: Ministry of Education

[9] IMH: Institute of Mental Health

MK

Yeah. People are self-diagnosing themselves. People are saying that they're depressed just from reading articles online, even though they're not necessarily clinically diagnosed.

Patrick

It's difficult to say whether it really is. There's a stigma, that's why a lot of people go to private clinics, psychiatrists, and counsellors at the heartlands. The first point of contact for the heartlanders is usually the family service centres and counselling services. I have one in my area, Whispering Hearts, that's usually the first point of contact. The other points of contact would be child guidance clinics and local polyclinics because now they have IMH expertise across the healthcare system in the hospitals as well as the polyclinics. So, you have that community care without having the stigma of going to IMH. Sometimes people are hesitant to admit that they need treatment and medication because of stigma. So, that in a nutshell encapsulates the different issues and challenges and the various interventions that come in. And it's not just one ministry, it is multi-ministry, because the issue cuts across different ages, different life stages—from the older folks who get dementia, Parkinson's, or depressive conditions, to the young who can suffer from bullying, cyberbullying, and even exposure to a lot of unclassified stuff on the web.

MENTAL HEALTH OVER THE YEARS

MK

I'm very curious. Because you've played many roles throughout your career, you've seen people from various groups. I was just wondering, is there a difference in the stigmas around mental health, say nineteen years ago as compared to now?

Patrick

I think there's more awareness of mental health issues. Previously, everybody classified it as *oh, you're not well, go to IMH.* But now, people realize there's a whole spectrum. You have mild depressive behaviour disorders all the way to the full spectrum where you really need treatment, and even tranquillizers in some situations. The awareness has gone up, definitely. More people are seeking help, but maybe through other ways. Awareness is one thing. People like yourself advocating for mental health. Twenty years ago, this topic—

MK

Nobody talked about it!

Patrick

Yeah, nobody talked about it! Now, increasingly, even for the special needs disability sectors, same thing. Twenty years ago, people would say, *You're just mischievous, you're just not behaving right, you're naughty.* But now naughty has a different dimension. Some people are quiet, but quiet may not be a good thing. Today's 'quiet' may suggest some other challenges.

I think awareness in the last two decades has gone up quite significantly. Sources of help and advocacy have gone up as well. Now, you have family service centres in the heartlands . . . not professional care like IMH treatment, but at least there's a buffer with counsellors, psychiatrists, psychologists to actually give you that initial level support. But, if I may, I'd like to highlight some gaps.

First, we really don't know how to help them. Let's say I've got a resident who has severe depression. Well, there are no powers to ask her to seek help. We do a lot of counselling support, we try to get the community to encourage her, or speak to her family members, but some of them may not have family members. They may refuse care and treatment, so what can we do to help them, short of invading their privacy and their personal fundamental liberties? For example, for a person with paranoid schizophrenia, I'm trying to help her because she probably needs medication and treatment professionally with a medical doctor, but I have to skirt around the issue. But if she doesn't want to go, it stops there. Those with family, it's okay, we try to encourage family. And family members also have challenges because the person who is mentally unwell may not agree, or may not think that he or she is mentally unwell. I hope we can find some way to plug this gap because there's a lot of community support. Not everyone will listen to you, and technically there's no power. I mean, the police have power. If you get someone with disorderly behaviour, looking very mentally unsound, who is creating some publicly disorderly behaviour, we'll probably arrest that person and have him or her for one or two weeks at IMH to seek treatment, to do a medical assessment to see if he or she really has a mental health condition. After that, if they find it's not really severe, there's no charge and the person is just released and goes back into the community and it's a vicious cycle. You don't solve the root problem. So, these are some of the frustrations.

MK

斩草除根 (To solve a problem, we must cut it at its roots). In Chinese we learnt that.

Patrick Tay

斩草不除根，春风吹又生 (If the root of a problem is not resolved, the problem will arise again at a later time).

PRE-EMPLOYMENT, IN-EMPLOYMENT, AND LEAVING EMPLOYMENT

MK

Since you talked about the workplace, let's zoom in a little bit about workers, because in your current role, one of the things you mentioned is that part of your responsibility and commitment is to ensure that the mental health of the workers is taken care of. So, what are some of the gaps or stigmas that are occurring in the workforce?

Patrick

Let's look at the three groups. Entry into employment, already in employment, and those leaving employment. Leaving employment could be retirement or retrenchment.

I'll start with leaving first. Leaving is for those who are retired. That's why you'll notice a lot of active ageing in the heartlands, because once they retire, what's next? When you're in a very high-strung, high-tempo kind of work, which many Singaporeans are in, and suddenly you stop, that's where the worries start. Self-worth and esteem issues will come up, especially if you don't already have a close network of friends, family members, and community. So that's why, if you noticed, we have set up a couple of active ageing and support activities in the heartlands. Of course, they're now unfortunately in a very low-touch, distanced way. So that's one part—when they leave the workforce altogether, whether it's voluntary or involuntary. That's why during the Circuit Breaker[10] period last year, when there were very few open spaces, and we couldn't do a lot of grassroot activities, the situation exacerbated. The feedback we got when we visited the old folks was, '*Eh wah*, I used to meet my friends every day, even for a brisk walk, now everything stopped, *leh*.' So, we don't know what's happening to them. They may go downhill, and therefore the need to resume. We're resuming in small ways now to stay occupied. You can't just be sitting there watching Netflix or doing nothing at home. So that's one—that's the leaving.

For those in employment, it's to create a support network and safe workplace. There are softer measures, the progressive

[10] Circuit Breaker refers to the three-month nationwide lockdown in Singapore to curb the spread of COVID-19.

measures, the work-life balance, the flexible work arrangements, so that your workplace can be somewhere that is supportive of whatever that you are facing because you could be looking after elderly parents, or child-bearing enrichments, or other exacting challenges. So, it's important for in-employment persons to have the support networks and also the proper human resources practices to help workers stay engaged and emotionally healthy. Supervisors play a very important role in detecting these issues because the staff themselves may not even realize that they've been working so hard. They may think they're doing great, but they don't realize they're going downhill emotionally and mentally.

For the pre-employment ones, it would be discriminatory practices. It's a very tight labour market in Singapore. I think employers are ready to hire any Singaporean if you have the necessary skills and experience. But the challenge is, *What if they had a previous mental health record?* And in most pre-employment medical checkups and surveys, they'll ask you this question, on the pretext that you're medically fit to do the job. We can understand this, for certain sectors that are very high-strung. For example, if you're working for the police, you're carrying firearms, so you can't have someone who's bordering on mental health issues for the safety of others, not so much anything else. There are specific jobs where it's understandable that some may not be suitable for the job. But I've also seen those who have recovered from depression assimilating into a new job very smoothly. So, it's about learning the best practices, the success cases, and finding the critical success factors to see how we can ensure that these job placements are as seamless as possible, and without discriminatory practices. This is my reading on the market and where the gaps are.

MK

Where do you think we're heading in terms of mental health with regards to the current group of workers in our society right now, in relation to the technological trends and advances that are happening in our world?

Patrick

Two things. With technological advances, digitalization and everything else, I'm sure there are some useful AI and systems that can help with the prevention and detection of mental health issues. Unfortunately, it's quite intrusive and borders on privacy issues. But if we can apply these technologies to track your rate of activity, attention span, fatigue levels, we will be able to raise awareness of these things that people can take note of. But between prevention and detection, prevention is important because that's where we can implement progressive practices in workplaces to ensure people stay engaged but don't lose focus, go off track, and get burnt out. The detection by supervisors and even AI systems could be helpful. *Why has this person been staring out the window for the last six hours?* Things like that. If you look at it, the sky's the limit.

Well, within current technology and resources, I think you can see a lot of focus on prevention and detection through other means. Like I said, for the elderly, we have created a very active engaged community that allows us to tap on communal support to detect issues in the community. You have mutual friends in the community, so you go for breakfast together or you go for brisk walks together. You can ask each other, *Are you all right or not? You look a bit dazed, are you okay?* That's the community detection capability. In terms of prevention, we have been doing a lot of community work with the regional healthcare cluster because the Health Promotion Board is very involved. MSF[11] is also very involved. In fact, schools are on it as well. The school counsellors and teachers have sort of a primer or training to

[11] MSF: Ministry of Social and Family Affairs

detect such signs and symptoms. Teachers now have private time with each and every student in the morning to ask the right questions, for example, *How are you feeling today? How do you find school work? Do you do a lot of tuition?* To kind of like suss out whether the person is a bit more stressed out, or perhaps hiding something, like being victims of bullying.

CATCHING ON TO THE CHANGES IN THE JOB MARKET

MK

You know, one of the things that I thought about is that, with all these technological advances, AI and all, a lot of people's jobs are going to get replaced, which means that unemployment rate is going to go up, which means more and more people are going to *zuobo*[12], and we talked about that just now.

Patrick

Yeah. We did some analysis locally, and frankly, I always say this line: *Whatever they can digitalize, mechanize, and robotize, will be digitalized, mechanized, and robotized.* So that's what the Industry Transformation Programme that came out in 2016 aimed to do: identify the jobs that would be replaced, or should I say, made redundant. We did some deep analysis across twenty-three different clusters and sectors.

The financial sector is a super digitalized area. Everything is a robotic process, automated on digital platforms. We're now in the fourth industrial revolution. If you noticed, whether it's the first, second, third, or fourth, the total number of net jobs in the world has never really gone down. It's ever increasing because as new industries emerge, there are new demands.

---

[12] Zuobo: Singapore slang for having nothing to do

So, how do we tilt the balance so that we have more new jobs than those that are disappearing? I think that awareness of disruption is very high. It's about 80 to 90 per cent. It's about how to make sure that people pick up the necessary skills and training so that they can segue into these new jobs. Some are transformed jobs. Meaning, if you used to be customer service, now you have a robot that answers customer queries. But because you have twenty years of experience, you're the one training the robots, which are only as good as the person keying in the replies. It's not so intuitive yet to judge people's feelings and why they ask certain questions. You can expect a lot of new and transformed jobs. Fortunately, in Singapore, our labour market is very tight. We have an ageing population and one of the lowest fatality rates in the world. I think even though we're in a downturn, there are still more jobs *vis-à-vis* the number of people looking for jobs.

If you look at very strict numbers based on the Industry Transformation Map projections and what is available currently in the labour market, the number of people who will be entering the labour market, and the labour force size—there isn't a shortage of jobs. I can't say this for the rest of the world, it's only for Singapore. For the rest of the world, you're right, it may be a challenge.

MK

How do you think we can bridge this gap since this is not going to be an issue in Singapore? That means the only issue here is our interest and openness to trying new things. Oftentimes, we like to be in our comfort zone.

Patrick

So therefore, the mindset change is going to be the most important—the mindset changes of the Tripartite Partners.

That means employers must be open to training their people and realize that these days, you cannot find a plug-and-play job function. Nobody will come in and be 100 per cent fit for your job. They'll probably be 50 to 60 per cent fit. Then you train them, you nurture them. That's why we have a lot of apprenticeships in the SG United Traineeship programme—so that the employer can find the right employee. Employees' mindset must change as well to be open, because frankly, some jobs have really disappeared, some jobs have really transformed, and there are new jobs. So be open about it. Give it a shot. You never know, you might like it. Just like in today's newspaper, this SQ[13] cabin crew stewardess, forty years old, was featured. After March last year, she started working in Khoo Teck Puat Hospital.

Then she realized, actually it is quite okay. I think the fact that she was open to it and realized that she had very adjacent transferable skills like dealing with customers, and now, patients, opened up a lot of possibilities. IT, healthcare, and community care services are hiring very aggressively, so the mindset of employers, mindset of employees, and in certain parts of the world, the mindset of the government as well must change. In Singapore, we're very fortunate, because there is a lot of support for worker training, so when you go for training, you don't have to worry.

MK

Got it. Is there anything else you want to say to people with regards to mental health and the work that they do? As there is a very strong correlation between mental health and work.

Patrick

For the community, I think one of the key things is that *no man is an island.* There is a lot of community support. The challenge is

---

[13] SQ refers to Singapore Airlines

whether you're willing to take the bold step to be open about it and to seek out some of this help and support. You have to take the first step. It's good to get professional help, and sometimes, you may not even know that you're bordering on mental health issues, so it's good to seek help and stay connected to people around you. Sometimes the best assessment is not by yourself, but by the people around you. So that's at a community level.

At the workplace level, we talked about recruitment, in-employment and when they leave their jobs. For those who are recruiting, my call is that even though a potential job applicant may have mental health issues, it's good to be open about it and see how we can consider them as potential job applicants. So be open about it and avoid discriminatory practices. At an entry-level and in-employment level, HR as well as employers and line supervisors need to be more aware of their employee's mental wellbeing and regulate arrangements. Particularly now in COVID, post COVID, the new normal, we're always online. But you can't really tell whether a person is well when online. It's good to have some micro-engagements. Lastly, those people who leave, post-retirement, I encourage everyone to stay connected. Stay connected to the community, stay active. For those who have left their jobs, we hope that companies in the outplacement process support these workers who are outplaced. There are a lot of schemes available, and I know a lot of employers do provide very strong support counselling measures post retrenchment. These are some of the actions we can take.

CHAPTER 4

The Complexities of Mental Health in the Workplace

By Serene Seng, Conscious Business Consultant, and Speaker, Senserene Pte Ltd

This extensive conversation looked into the multiple ways employers and employees are challenged by workplace norms. On an organizational level, Serene Seng pointed out that CEOs and managers sometimes do not hold the absolute power to create change, and yet the responsibility to protect the mental health and wellbeing of employees still lie with the organization at large. Especially during these uncertain times, leaders must still be able to provide direction and an overarching vision for their team members. While leaders may strive to be a role model and set a good example for their team, they often have to grapple with their own struggles as well. It is this complex set of dynamics that makes mental health in the workplace a very difficult landscape to navigate in a pandemic and post-pandemic world.

OUR PROPENSITY TO PRETEND THAT EVERYTHING IS FINE

Serene

The work that I do is all about mental health, and I do it because I feel that the priority now is mental health at the workplace. It was very tough in 2020, not just in Singapore, but worldwide. I think on some level, people are expected by their organizations to function as normal, to go back to work as normal, when the world is no longer normal.

I don't know how you feel, but I feel there's too much emphasis on the company going back to normal. Granted we're no longer under lockdown and we don't *have* to be working from home, which is good. But there's just too much emphasis on *hey, we should just go back to normal*, and I'm just wondering if we are even ready.

MK

Not just physically, but also emotionally and mentally, which is an equation that is oftentimes not mentioned in the economic sense. Because . . . I mean, think about it this way. For most of us, our understanding of emotions is weak and vague to begin with. We were not trained in school to deal with the complexity of our emotions.

Serene

Next week, I'm interviewing a psychiatrist[14] from IMH[15] and I'm going to ask him, are we normal? Are we back to normal yet? Like what's the situation here from what IMH can see?

---

[14] Workplace Mental Health in Singapore interview: https://www.youtube.com/watch?v=E5Q_A_0O4TM

[15] IMH: Institute of Mental Health (Singapore's only hospital dedicated to mental health)

MK

What do you think? Are we going back to normal?

Serene

I think there's a lot of sweeping stuff under the carpet. We're pretending that nothing has changed.

And one of the issues we don't address is that there are so many levels to workplace mental health. I do a weekly live interview series on workplace mental health[16] with people from all walks of life, from business leaders, to people who are coaches, to those who run the workplace mental health programmes for the whole country, and everything in between. What I'm hearing from all levels is that there are so many minute aspects of the situation that we are not looking into. The biggest one, in terms of work, is that work is no longer what it used to be, but nobody knows what is in front of them because there have been so many changes in the last one year that nobody actually dares to say what this year will be like. Honestly, nobody dares to say.

I sympathize with them, but we can't just sit here and do nothing. I mean, I don't know what's happening any more than anyone does, but I cannot just tell my people, *We don't know what's happening and we don't know what we're going to do.* We have to give some kind of direction.

MK

Inspire vision, direction, hope, especially when you are a leader.

Serene

Yeah! As a leader, I still have to give directions to my people. I still must delegate work to my people. I still must tell my

[16] Workplace Mental Health (The Serene View live interview series), https://www.youtube.com/playlist?list=PLAjgsC420ch6RgT7l6vJyxd-6Vl9riQPC.

people what to do even when I don't know what to do. When I ask the guy above me, he also doesn't know, and I can tell he doesn't know. He's making it up and I'm making it up from his making it up, and I don't know who is on top of him who is also making it up!

MK

And then it becomes a vicious cycle. Nobody knows what the hell is going on. There's no clarity.

Serene

Yes, correct. So right now, based on my conversations with all those leaders, I think there's a whole spectrum of leaders. People who want to build a conscious business tend to be people who are aware and caring towards their people, so they actually do want to do something about it themselves. I can tell. The leader thinks, *My people are not doing well and I want to do something for them, but there are two issues. One, I'm struggling myself. Two, I don't know what is helpful.* What do you say to a person whose family is in another country, hospitalized and isolated from COVID, and she cannot go back? What do you say to that person?

I guess if you were to put it in a bland way, the crux of the issue is really about seeing people as people. Can we see them that way and reach out to them? When you get together with a stranger, you will realize that you have so much in common with them. You have so much commonality with them. There's a study they did where they got people to just stand there for, I think six minutes, looking into each other's eyes and doing nothing.[17] Don't say a word, don't do anything.

---

[17] Global Ethic Foundation, 'The Eye Contact Experiment', accessed on 23 August 2021, https://www.global-ethic.org/the-eye-contact-experiment/.

MK

Well, I did something similar too. That was one of our works in the exhibition called Connection Without Words. I first created it back in 2018, and I recreated it in 2020 to make it better. And what was interesting was that we got people from the deaf community to be part of the experience.

It was very powerful because one of the things I did was I isolated the people with normal hearing from their sense of hearing using headphones with a sound that takes them away from their normal senses, and got them to connect with each other so that they can start relating to each other more. I wouldn't have known about this if I didn't hang out with people in the deaf community, but I realized that there's so much stigma out there that if we're not in their shoes, we wouldn't know what exactly they're dealing with. And it's not a coincidence that their self-esteem and self-confidence are affected, and that they're also so guarded, because they don't feel like they're part of anything. That's why our exhibition is called *Threading Worlds*. Part of it is about bringing different worlds together—whether it's the blind, the deaf, the wheelchair-bound, or the palliative, to come together. Because we are all human beings.

Serene

But Singapore is very conformist, and as a result, we have a natural aversion to being non-conforming. For example, if you notice, you seldom see the intellectually disabled in public. I have friends whose kids are intellectually disabled or autistic. The way that people look at those kids makes their parents not want to bring them out because, *Why should I subject them to this kind of discrimination*? I think because Singapore has such a great need for conformity, discrimination is even worse in Singapore. Because everybody's like *must score well, my kid's so clever*. If you're intellectually disabled, or you're autistic, you have to deal with a lot of stigma. And can you imagine mental disorders as well? If you have a kid with a mental disorder, same thing.

It's one thing to say, *Oh, we're very harmonious, different races get together very well.* True, but the flip side of this conformism is that if you don't belong in the in-group, then we don't treat you very well any more. And you'd be surprised—even my Indian or Malay friends tell me that they feel discrimination despite decades of education on racial harmony. They still feel that way. And if you go out to restaurants and look at the people sitting at the tables, they tend to be racially divided.

MK

There are so many issues that people don't want to deal with, so they keep sweeping them underneath the carpet. And when we do that, what we don't realize is that whatever we don't want to deal with, it compounds, it accumulates. The problem is how long does it last before the tank is fully filled and it erupts?

Serene

I honestly think in Singapore, we have a great propensity for pretending that nothing's wrong. I don't know whether you take public transport, but the next time you do, take the train and do something unusual. It can be anything. Just stand up on the chair. Just stand there calmly and quietly. You will realize that the entire carriage will ignore you. Everybody will act as if nothing has happened.

MK

They're all still in their own worlds on their phones.

Serene

I don't think they're in their own world. They know that you are standing on the chair. I think they've just been trained to *mind their own business.*

MK

Interesting.

Serene

I'm sure as you're growing up, your parents will tell you this: *mind your own business.*

MK

Yes, mind your own business. Sounds very familiar!

Serene

People can take care of themselves, right? Whatever is happening, they can take care of themselves. It's not your problem so don't meddle. They have been trained that way for twenty years. If you've been trained that way for twenty years, what happens when somebody stands on a chair? As long as he's not threatening me, he seems to be fairly safe, okay, fine, just leave him to do his own thing. And the thing is, I will tell you this as a Singaporean, it is something that I love. Because it allows me to do all kinds of things in my daily life, and I know that no one will come and bother me, no one will threaten me, no one will do anything to me. In many parts of the world, if you do something like that, somebody will come and threaten you, like *get down* or *I will do something to you.* But in Singapore, nothing will happen to you. People will just go on as normal.

I mean, I love that because I'm the kind of person who will go to a park and start dancing without music and nobody cares!

But on the other hand, if you need help, then you have to be thick-skinned enough to go and talk to somebody. And you have to be very persistent because the first thing they'll think is, *Is there a hidden camera? Are you trying to trick me?*

MK

Or are you trying to get something out of me? We have a very transactional, utilitarian mentality.

Serene

Correct. And actually, I don't think Singaporeans are not compassionate. I mean, look at all the amount of donations that people give whenever something happens. People are very compassionate. I think we are comfortable, and when people are comfortable, they have the capacity to give, but at the same time, they've also been taught that other people can take care of themselves. *If it's not your business, don't meddle: you're bothering them.* They will never go and say, 'Are you all right? Are you okay?' There are countries that run these campaigns. UK[18] has it, Australia[19] has it—the 'Are You Okay' campaign. If this campaign runs in Singapore, it's just going to fail massively because A, I won't ask you, '*Are you okay*,' and B, even if I ask you, what's your reaction? '*I'm okay, never mind, don't worry, don't worry!*' You'll just fail massively because we've all been taught, 'Don't bother other people, people can take care of their own business!'

I don't think Singaporeans are cold or emotionless. I know we top the world survey for being emotionless,[20] but I don't actually think that we are. I think that Singaporeans are fairly compassionate. But at the same time, we also feel that we shouldn't bother people. People should be fine. The assumption is that you should be all right. I shouldn't come and ask you if you're all right as if I feel that you're not all right—

---

[18] See Me Scotland, 'Campaigns and Activities', accessed on 23 August 2012, https://www.seemescotland.org/workplace/tackling-discrimination-at-work/campaigns-and-activities/.

[19] R U OK, 'R U OK', accessed on 23 August 2021, https://www.ruok.org.au/.

[20] Jon Clifton, 'Singapore Ranks as Least Emotional Country in the World', Gallup, 21 November 2012, https://news.gallup.com/poll/158882/singapore-ranks-least-emotional-country-world.aspx.

MK

And I'm making you not all right.

Serene

Yeah, correct, so there's that thinking. People tend to just ignore it. If you do anything weird, they'll just ignore. And seriously, for years, I loved it. I would never go and live in a country like America, where everybody comes and asks you how you are. I'm like, 'Leave me alone!'

[laughter]

So I love Singapore. But on the other hand, if you're talking about mental health, it's not a very conducive environment. It's not surprising that anxiety and depression are the top two mental disorders in Singapore.[21]

Look at it this way, if you're depressed, what do you do? You shut down. You shut yourself in your room. You don't want to eat. You don't want to sleep. You don't want to do anything. You don't want to engage in life any more. Right? Who's going to help you, given the Singaporean mentality? I mean, even if you huddle in a corner of the train, they'll also feel, *Okay, never mind, maybe they need some space*. That's why these things persist. Add to that the fact that anxiety is an extension of our national tendency towards *kiasu*-ism. *Kiasu, kiasi, kiamsiap, kanchiong*[22]—which one has got nothing to do with anxiety? If you push kiasu-ism to the max, what you get is a GAD, right? Generalized Anxiety Disorder.

And it's very interesting because the same group of parents who will get their kids to compete with other kids in school, will

---

[21] Ministry of Health, 'What Are The Demographics Of Patients Receiving Psychiatric Treatment And Mental Health Support', 6 January 2020, https://www.moh.gov.sg/news-highlights/details/what-are-the-demographics-of-patients-receiving-psychiatric-treatment-and-mental-health-support.

[22] Kiasu, kiasi, kiamsiap, kanchiong: Singapore slangs which denote the varying degrees of anxiety and paranoia that Singaporeans often experience collectively as a culture.

probably jump into the pool to save those other kids. But in school, you must be the best. So where do all these contradictions come in? When I look at the Singaporean character, I think we're very interesting people. Very conformist, but at the same time, very complaintive. Compassionate, but at the same time, competitive, right? Can't be bothered, but at the same time, we will STOMP[23] each other for small things.

And I don't know if you believe in this, but when I was in Australia, they told me that if you come from a country where there's a lot of land and there's a great expanse, like in Australia where you can drive for a whole day and you'll never see a single person—no person, no building—your character will be more open and expansive. But if you come from a place where everything is very cramped, then people become pettier. And I'm like, maybe.

MK

It may have to do with the spaces that we live in, because that physical space is also a reflection of our psychological space as well.

Serene

Yeah, but that's what the Australians told me. I mean, they're really very chill. Small things don't bother them. If you overtake people on the road, it doesn't matter. If you overtake people on the road here, people get very outraged. I'm like, why is it that small things like these matter so much to us? And maybe it's the physical space.

MK

And we operate on the scarcity mentality.

[23] STOMP is a citizen journalism website, which is often used by Singaporeans for highlighting socially unacceptable behaviour exhibited in public.

Serene

And it is true, right? We're running out of space. We have a scarcity mentality because we don't have enough space. We feel that we're running out of space. We live in the most expensive city in the world.[24] We're running out of money. Is it wrong for Singaporeans to have a scarcity mentality? I don't think so. I think our standard of living has gone down since the 90s. People may not be consciously aware of it, but subconsciously they're aware: *Hey, it's getting harder and harder to live the same kind of life.* If you look at the lower middle-income group, for them to make ends meet, it's getting harder and harder.

MK

There's a lot of survival conversations, a lot of talk about getting a good job so that we don't have to worry about rainy days. The lower-income group thinks about it differently, the middle-income group thinks about it differently, and the upper-income group thinks about it differently as well. There are different frameworks based on socioeconomic status.

'IF I WORK HARD, I WILL ACHIEVE A BETTER FUTURE.' IS IT TRUE?

Serene

One of the things I've been worried about for quite a few years, and been talking to different people about, is this. You see, Singapore is built on the basis that people believe, 'If I work hard,

---

[24] Economist Intelligence Unit, 'Worldwide Cost of Living 2020: How is Covid-19 affecting the prices of consumer goods?', accessed on 23 August 2021, https://www.eiu.com/topic/worldwide-cost-of-living (Singapore is ranked most expensive city in the world from 2014-2019 in the Worldwide Cost of Living Survey published by The Economist Intelligence Unit).

I will achieve a better future for myself and my family.' My belief however, is that if I put in effort, I may not become the best of the best—

MK

If I do my work, I'll be rewarded, and therefore, my life would be better.

Serene

Correct. If I put in the effort, I'll have the opportunity to get a better life for myself and my children. Actually, I think the whole of Singapore is built on this one basis. And it was true for many years. My parents were born poor and built their own wealth, and my grandparents were immigrants who built a new life here. But now, is that still true? Let's say you're in the lower middle-income group, and you may have graduated from ITE[25] because your family wasn't able to send you to a top pre-school. For the last twenty years, you've not had that competitive privilege, and now you've graduated from ITE. And you come from a family where both of your parents work daily wages. What is the belief system of somebody like that? Do they still believe that *if I work hard, I will be able to gain a better future for myself and my kids?* And if not, what's going to happen to Singapore? Because it's a pyramidal system. There are always fewer rich than poor. If the bottom half of the people lose hope that *I can get a better future for myself*—what's going to happen to society?

And I tell you honestly, when I speak to a lot of these kids now, I don't see the same sense of hope for the future that my parents had, or even we had. When I graduated, I truly believed that if I worked hard, I could get a good future for myself, and so did my friends. Everybody believed that we could go to university

[25] ITE: Institute of Technical Education

and we could get a job. But the kids nowadays, even if they work very hard, from ITE they go to polytechnic, from polytechnic they go to university, could they get a better job, a better future? These kids are not stupid; you think they don't know this? Why do you think so many of them are becoming YouTubers and influencers? Because they know. They know as well as I do that you can get a degree, a PhD, but is that still a competitive advantage in the workplace? I have seen this trend, probably for like five or six years now, at the very least from the beginning of the last recession. A lot of people lost their jobs and couldn't climb back up again. And then you look at it and ask yourself, what about the kids nowadays? When they graduate, how do they feel? And if you have this issue, what's going to happen next? What's going to happen to Singapore over the next ten years? I don't know. I can only tell my own child, 'Make your plans: you may not be staying here for the rest of your life.' I've been here all my life, but do I expect my kid to be here? I don't know. My biggest fear for Singapore has got nothing to do with politics or education. I really feel that our Gini coefficient has gone up crazily over the last twenty years. Now the rich are so rich, but the poor are getting poorer. Now we're even starting welfare for the poor—medical, income, things like that. But is that enough?

MK

Is that enough, and when will it be enough?

Serene

I think however much we give . . . You know the basis of welfare, right? Welfare creates dependency. No amount of welfare that you give can replace the hope that *if I work hard, I can make things better for myself.* If you ask me whether I'm worried about Singapore, that's the biggest one. The rest I think we can solve.

MK

Got it. This is very powerful.

HOW DO ORGANIZATIONAL STRUCTURES AFFECT MENTAL HEALTH IN THE WORKPLACE?

MK

When we talk about workplace mental health, there are a few things I want to look at. I just want to state the context of where I'm coming from. I come from a space where I'm a trained life coach. I do a lot of performance coaching and creative coaching with the corporate workplace environment as well. But I think right now, a lot of people are expecting the company to do certain things for them. For example, people are requesting that they should permanently work from home. I feel that there are a few layers we have to look at. We need to recognize that it is fundamentally the responsibility of the individuals to make sure that their mental health is taken care of. What do I mean by that? As much as we're looking at the different layers from the organizational level, fundamentally, we have to recognize that the ownership still lies with the individual and what the individual wants to do about it. And again, we're talking about personal mental health, and we need to start looking into those factors as well.

Serene

Well, I can tell you that. I am a management consultant, and we take care of organizational development. Actually, why don't you tell me what you think, because I think I've been in this space for too long. I have a lot of my own, for lack of a better word, my sacred cows, and so I don't think it's useful for me to say anything at this point in time. So why don't you go ahead?

MK

Got it. So, on the individual, again, we're talking about individual's responsibility towards mental health. But I think the other aspect we need to look at in terms of organizational structure is, how can we create more effective structures for people in the company to thrive? A lot of times, people need to find a place in the company where they can really contribute in terms of their skills, their talents, and even their gifts as well. And for them to find that spot, part of it is about creating an ecosystem that allows people to perform in their own ways, whatever that means, because everybody's definition of performance is different. If we can create a structure that allows that kind of freedom for people to express their performance in the way that they want, that will definitely give them a boost, because when people do the things they love, they perform better, which also means higher results.

A lot of people think that burnout happens because of the imbalances in their work life, such as the work hours and job scope. But truthfully, from my experiences, it's not really the case. It's because there is a misalignment with what they're doing, or even their job as a whole. That sucks away a lot of their energy and life force and as a result, they get tired and exhausted before long because they're not able to confront or overcome whatever they have to deal with.

If you have strong alignment towards your job, even with these imbalances, you will still be able to thrive. And furthermore, these imbalances are often created from the imbalances in a person's internal state in the first place. In coaching, we look into what is causing the imbalance within the person. Oftentimes, the real issue that is underlying is something deeper in themselves, which has got nothing to do with the organization in the first place.

Then the other aspect we also need to look at is culture. Now, when I say culture, I'm talking about whether the environment, the culture, the ecosystem in the company, and the organization as a whole, facilitates the growth and development of a person. But, as a matter of fact, organizational interests always come first before individual interests. Because in organizations, there are certain structures, and certain people who need to be in that hierarchy. I think this is something that individuals have to recognize as well—the organization's goals and objectives always come first before the individual. The only thing the organization can do is create a constant and strong alignment between their goals and the individual's goals as well. Because if that alignment exists, there's a lower chance for people to burn out.

Now, in the job that we do, there are things that we love, and there are also things that we don't love. And I think part of the equation is about how individuals can avoid sacrificing different parts of their identity in order to fit into the role they're supposed to play. Are there ways that individuals can remain authentic in what they do because they come from a space of love and alignment?

Serene

How do you think leaders can enable that? Let's go with your presumption, which is we're in a company where the company's goals take precedence over mine; where the culture is, I wouldn't say toxic, but it's business as usual, profits first, bottom line first; where I am in a job for which I am reasonably suited, and I won't say completely misaligned to, but it's a job. And I'm not overly oppressed or anything. We come to this question: *How do I not lose pieces of my identity that are equally important to me?* Even though I need the job, and it's 2021. People are being retrenched. It's not like I can just walk off and find an ideal job. It's not a horrible job. But if I am your leader, what do I do?

MK

I think we live in a world of constant negotiation. Part of aligning ourselves to the organization's goals is also a negotiation. It's also about the discernment of the roles that you signed up for and the roles that you are being paid for. Now, a lot of times misalignments happen because of different expectations. Person A expects this, whereas the reality offers another kind of event that creates a mismatch. That mismatch creates problems. If the person doesn't address it or clear it up with whoever they are reporting to in the organization, it creates a problem. Part of it is really about that self-awareness, where they clear it up the moment they have the awareness that there's a certain misalignment. But of course, certain roles, like that of a politician or even a leader in the organization, don't necessarily allow a person to do that kind of clearing. Even if they're misaligned, they have to literally mask it up. Because they're expected to do so in that role itself.

For example, the manager usually won't go and tell others about what they feel. I mean, if the job of the manager is to manage, they won't usually tell the subordinates their own personal misalignment with the organization unless they have a personal relationship to begin with. That masking up is oftentimes very easy at the start. But the act of masking up also creates a lot of problems down the road. Does it make sense?

Serene

Makes sense.

MK

Okay, so let me just answer your question. In terms of what leaders can do specifically, I think besides creating a culture, leaders have to be aware of where their people are at and create a system for their managers to operate from. The question is, can misalignments be detected at an early stage? The answer is yes, but oftentimes in corporate organizations, by the time people realize that, it's too late already. People already have an exit plan. So, part of it is creating a structure that allows them to build stronger relationships with one another. It's a people game, because if the relationships are strong, when there are misalignments, the employees know that they are able to reach out to their employers, their managers, and leaders, with an open heart. And I think that's very well missing in the corporate structure.

Serene

I've been doing this for fifteen years. To me, the problem is very simple. If you are hurt, you can go off and get yourself healed. But if you go back to the work environment where you will be hurt again, then no amount of self-healing is going to solve the problem. In terms of physical health, I think workplaces have more advanced protocols. But in terms of mental health, I don't think there's that. I feel that to expect a worker to take responsibility for their mental health, which is what you've asserted, is as unreasonable as expecting a chimney sweeper working in Britain in the 1800s to take care of their physical health because when you look at the power differential, who has the power?

MK

The organization.

Serene

To say, *Hey, it's your job, mental health is your personal responsibility, you should look after yourself. You have already been hurt by your childhood and that is the reason you're reacting this way,* and so on. I will tell you honestly, from a practitioner point of view, it's not an acceptable excuse.

To me, as organizations, businesses do have power. One of my beliefs is that when you have power, you have the responsibility to ensure that you are not abusing this power on those who are, shall we say, more disadvantaged than you are. And if you look at an organization versus an average worker—we're not talking about C-suite or anything like that, just the average run-of-the-mill employee—I think it'll be hard to argue that the employee has any power other than to walk away from that organization. So, when you look at an issue as a system rather than an isolated problem, what you will see is that systematically, we have come from a different place.

I will put it this way: companies were set up initially for purely profit-driven concerns. And in social development, global development, we have not had this concern for the individual, concern for the different aspects of humans, as we have had over the last 200 years. I would say we had it in the ancient past, and we've lost it, and now we're trying to recover it. So, organizations are still built to get the most profit, not to get the best out of people. And in the first, maybe even second industrial age, that made sense, right? Because if you're a production worker, the longer you sit in your chair, the faster I can push the conveyor belt past you, the more widgets you put into the circuit, the more money I make, regardless of the cost to you as an individual. But as we move into the fourth—and some people argue that we're in the fifth—industrial age, knowledge work is becoming more important because AI will ultimately replace all of the routine work. The only value humans will have is in creative problem solving, innovation, and human relationships. And all of those involve the capacity of the mind that cannot be pushed simply by saying, *I want you to meet these expectations.* If I say, *I want you to meet five times more people to close more sales*, does that truly benefit the company, or is it more beneficial to meet fewer people but build a stronger relationship with them?

MK

It's very hard for us to just say yes or no, because it really depends on the contexts, the circumstances, where the organizations are at, and also the skills and development of the individuals. Many factors.

Serene

Exactly. With knowledge work, volume, time spent at work, productivity—when measured traditionally, which is number of tasks per hour—is no longer the most value-adding, and is no longer the right way to measure a person's contribution or value to the company. But as a whole, whether it is in terms of our organizational structures, our compensation and benefit systems, or performance management systems, we have not moved to that stage yet. And because we have not moved to that stage yet, what you are seeing is this misalignment. A misalignment of what a worker truly needs to do and the structures that are set up to enable that work.

And so, when I say that that's probably the biggest price that organizations pay in workplace mental health right now, that's what I mean. Because we have just had a pandemic, and in many countries, it's not *just had*, it's *are having*. And what you will see is companies still expect people to go to work as usual, do business as usual, accomplish your tasks as usual. If all I needed to do was put a widget into the circuit, sure, that still can be done. But if I need to do complex problem solving and your mind is—

MK

Doesn't have the space for it.

Serene

Correct. And it's a knowledge economy that we're moving towards. Most of us are doing knowledge work. And in knowledge work, I would argue that rest and the ability to take a step back and put together your ideas is even more important than the time you spend working. Newton didn't get his ideas from being at his desk; he got it from resting under a tree. Archimedes got it from taking a bath. Your best ideas come to you not when you're hard at work. If you look at the way companies are moving at the moment, I will say that yes, they are responsible, but as you've also noted, because they have the power and the privilege in that way, the chances of them voluntarily changing are not high.

We're down to two things. One, just as in the case of chimney sweepers in the past, workers will have to refuse to take jobs that endanger their mental health. Given the current economic climate and given the current power differential, I don't see that as being possible in the near future. Instead, people are dropping out, which is why there's a rise in the gig economy, especially among younger people, because they are looking at what companies are offering and going, *No, I'm not buying this transaction any more, and I'm stepping away from this.* That's a choice that, increasingly, young people are making. I actually applaud them for it. I know a lot of Gen-Xers have apprehension about this behaviour because we have had to slog it out, but I don't wish that to be the reality for every coming generation. I don't wish that. I truly wish upon them fulfilling work and the sort of work-rest cycle that is mentally healthy, even though we never had it as kids. I think it is mean of us to say that just because we never had a chance to have it, you guys cannot have it. I salute them for making the call. Now, people in my generation can't. We have too many responsibilities, and we've invested too much in the game to be able to walk away. But I think that change is coming, and organizations will be wise to recognize it. Because, ultimately, the people aged forty to sixty will exit the workforce in the next twenty years, and the world will be the world of millennials. The companies that won't recognize their demands are just not going to continue to exist, that's all. And I think that's a good change for business.

The second one which is a little bit what I'm pushing you for is that, the fact of the matter is, we're still here, now. It's not twenty years down the road yet. I'll tell you, I've met enough CEOs to know that even the CEO doesn't have complete power to change. There's no magic set of leaders who can do that, but what I was going to say is that if let's say I'm a line manager. I recognize the issue, and I want to address it. What do I do? And actually, these are the people who are coming forth with focus. *What do I do? I know that this is a problem, I do want to do something about it, but my organization is not going to change.* I will not say that we work for some slave-driving corporation, but let's say it's an average organization. They're not particularly wonderful, but they're not terribly bad. *What do I do? What can I do to protect my people, to enable them to thrive, within the scope of my authority?* And that's where I'm really coming at when I'm talking to you, because I don't think you have experience changing organizations, but I think that you've worked with many leaders, and you've helped them. And I'm sure among the stuff you've helped them with, there'll be issues around *how do I better manage my people?*

MK

Yep.

Serene

And so, what have you found that is helpful? What have you found that is *oh no, don't go there, even though it sounds good; just don't go there, it's terrible.* What are the landmines, what are the benefits?

MK

I think to follow whatever I shared with you earlier on, individuals have to recognize that they have a part to play. I'm not saying that corporates should not do more. I think both should run at equal pace as well. When individuals do their part, they become stronger in their foundations, and in terms of the core corners of their mental health, emotional health, and physical health as well. This will enable them to make better choices and have the clarity that they need to get things done. Basically, the heart, body, and mind are aligned. When I talk about alignment, I come from that space. And I totally get where you're coming from in terms of what the organizations can do more.

I'll just speak from my personal experience in terms of what I hear and see. I think a lot of leaders struggle to build the culture and ecosystem that they desire when they first set up the whole business. And it's always the culture not being the right fit for people that causes them to leave. Besides the job, the environment also plays a huge part in whether the individual holds on to their job, because the environment holds them. Then the question is, how can we create a more conscious environment, knowing that a lot of the current practices have shown that the environment hasn't really been that successful at supporting people? It's not as easy to build as it sounds. People talk about the cultural codes within the work environment and all that, but there are distinctions. There's a difference between a culture and structure built for three people and one built for seven people. There's a difference between a culture and structure built for eleven people, for a hundred people, and a thousand people as well. So, part of it is about realigning the values. What does the company stand for? We need to look deeper into the vision and mission of the organization as well and examine how well the organization is living up to that. Does this make sense, Serene?

Serene

Yeah.

MK

A lot of times, people don't really reinvent their structure after they build culture and eventually, over time, things get messy. Actually, when it comes to cleaning up the organization from a structural point, people also need to go through a certain level of cleaning within themselves towards their relationship to the organization.

The clearing part is very important. The organization needs to create a safe space for people to do clearing, for people to be able to express what they're really feeling.

Serene

What do you mean by clearing?

MK

Any misalignments that they have towards the organization. Any misalignments that the organization has towards them.

For instance, I love my job, but you know, I don't like how the management runs the organization. I don't like how ineffective and inefficient it is. I don't like the delays in my pay, for example.

Serene

Are you talking about airing grievances?

MK

Yes, that's included as well. Things that require clearing are things that will cause grey areas within a person's relationship with the organization. The whole point of the clearing is to make sure that individuals get to express themselves to the organization, and from an organizational standpoint, they also have a space to express themselves to the individuals as well. Part of it also comes in the form of acknowledgement. Acknowledgement of what went well, what did not go so well, and what can be improved. Usually, when individuals do a clearing with the organization, it's coming from an emotional space more than anything else. It's really about clearing and sorting out these emotions instead of leaving them dangling. And if we were to look into the history of why this is important, it is simply because we have not been taught how to use our hearts to feel our whole lives.

Serene

Actually, I want you to elaborate on what you mean by organization, because there is obviously no way to do a clearing with the *organization*. The organization is an abstract concept.

MK

The general manager of the organization who represents the organization.

Serene

So, you're talking about the CEO?

MK

Correct.

Serene

So, you feel there should be a way for employees to directly reach and address their grievances with the CEO?

MK

Why not?

Serene

Well, I don't think it's a question of why not. It's a question of how we can make it possible, especially in larger organizations. The largest organizations in the world now number over 100,000 people. When you talk about the human capacity of a CEO—

MK

Okay, if you're talking about those kinds of numbers, then those CEOs must have leaders and managers that represent different regions to begin with. Then, these people can act as vessels for the organization.

Serene

Even if I give you a very small number, let's say 5,000 people. Is it possible to say that the CEO should be available to address the grievances of 5,000 people?

MK

It doesn't necessarily have to be the CEO, but it needs to be somebody who has the power to represent the organization.

Serene

Like who, the HR? CEO? Deputy CEO?

MK

Maybe, because different structures require different things. I can't really answer that. Certain structures operate from leaders, by training leaders in different regions. Whereas other organizations operate from whatever you just said, where they're run by managers, for example. Especially when the organization is so big, there's only so much that the CEO can do. Part of it is also the leadership structure that they need to have in the first place. When it comes to clearing, that clearing is to make sure that the people are clear towards the organization on an emotional level, on a mental level, and on a physical level as well. They need to sort out any misalignments and declare them to the organization rather than letting them spill over. Anything that is swept under the carpet or spilt over will always have a consequence in the relational line as well. Relationships have their own rules as well. Likewise, in emotions as well. That's why I emphasize the clearing. Of course, when the organization gets bigger and bigger and bigger, we need structures around that whereby people can sort that out directly with whoever is capable and equipped enough to represent the organization. It could even be the supervising officer that they report to. I feel the clearing part is missing, that's why I emphasize it.

Serene

Fair.

PRACTICING SELF-LOVE AND MASTERY AT WORK

MK

There's another question that I think will be interesting to discuss. How can individuals at the workplace, or even in their personal capacity, work deeper on their self-love? Because when we talk about mental health, self-love is an important part of the equation as well. What does it mean to take care of yourself?

Serene

I would say that a lot of my work is on systems and on an organizational level, so I do much less work on individuals. I do coach leaders, but the work I do with them is more focused on their teams.

MK

When you say coach, what do you mean?

Serene

I do executive coaching. I'm a Gallup Strengths Coach, I'm an ICF[26] PCC[27]-certified coach, and I'm also an Action Learning

---

[26] ICF: International Coaching Federation

[27] PCC: Professional Coaching Certification

coach, so I'm actually certified in quite a few modalities. And I got certified to be a Belbin Teams Coach.

MK

And you do a lot of profiling as well?

Serene

Yes, I do a lot of profiling. I'm also a Certified Saville Wave and MBTI[28] practitioner, so I definitely do a lot of profiling. I try to get people into the best job fit—we call this talent-job fit—to discover their greatest talent and then craft the job for them. I think it's quite different from what people think. A lot of people think *I have a job, then I find the best person to fit into that job.* But actually, what you have are tasks that need to be done, which we roughly group into jobs. But if you've ever worked in an organization, you'll notice that as time goes by, the work that you do and the tasks that you manage morphs, and what is written on paper in your job description may not necessarily be what you're doing. What happens then? My question is, why can people not do this at the start? Naturally, there's the issue of eligibility and suitability. Eligibility means you have the paper qualifications. For example, if you're an accountant, you need to have ACCA[29] qualifications. Suitability means you have the talent and innate strengths that allow you to shine at a job. That is the difference between being an outsourced accountant, an in-house accountant, or an auditor. All of these require ACCA qualifications but have very different job scopes.

So then, where would you really shine, and how can we bring on a person and then look at the job and, in some way, adapt the job to the person while keeping the outcomes constant?

[28] MBTI: Myers Briggs Type Indicator

[29] ACCA: Association of Chartered Certified Accountants

Because ultimately, does it matter how you do a job, as long as you achieve the outcomes that the company requires you to do? I often use the example of sales. A lot of people think sales require extroversion and talkativeness, but there are salespeople who are introverted, who do enormous amounts of research, and then present to other introverts with a great need for detail and close them that way. What I'm trying to say is, if your outcome is sales, you may not need to dictate the way the job is done.

And I think the next step would be for companies to think about what the outcomes are, not even out of a person, but out of a team. And where do I find a team? This is the reason I was so interested in getting certified in Belbin. Where do I find a team where the sum of the parts is greater than the whole? How do I get them together and allow them to, in a way, complement each other to such an extent that they're able to achieve all of these objectives and more? Bringing this idea forward, we come to what we call network organizations. I've been asking around whether there are any such organizations, and a very good friend of mine, a professor, says that Haier is currently doing it. You know the Chinese electronics company?

I will not say they are a perfect example of this, but this is what they're doing. They have small groups of people who are put together with complementary strengths and obviously with the knowledge, experience and skills needed to work on specific projects. Then they liaise with other groups. Why? Because human beings are, by nature, social animals. I think even the most introverted person requires some relationships. And we have found that nobody can be perfect: this is what we've always known, but a team can have complementary strengths such that they cover most, if not all, tasks. And so, that enables the team to be able to do much better work than just a single person, and it also enables people to build the kind of relationships that they need for support. Dan Pink was the one who talked about motivation at work.[30] We usually think of pay, workplace health and safety, and a generally pleasant physical environment when we think about workplace motivation. But it's like hygiene in COVID. If I'm not hygienic, I get sick, but if I'm extremely hygienic, it doesn't make me less sick. So, if you don't pay people enough, obviously, that is a big factor and people will go away, but if you pay people tons and tons, but don't look into the other factors that truly make people happy, the pay alone will not make them happy. Dan Pink said that what's needed is: autonomy, expertise, and relationships, if I'm not mistaken. Autonomy means I have control over my own work, whether it be authority, freedom, or whatever you call it; I have this control. Expertise is the ability to be the best at what I do, and this ties in with Gallup's research as well. Gallup's research is based on, *Do I have the opportunity every day to do what I'm best at?*[31] *So that I can develop my expertise, I can develop my mastery, I can become a master in something.*

MK

You're talking about being a master in their own personal—

Serene

No, to master certain tasks or areas of work.

MK

Yeah, correct. But it goes back to the individual's willingness to commit themselves to mastery.

---

30 Dan Pink, 'The puzzle of motivation', TED, July 2009, https://www.ted.com/talks/dan_pink_the_puzzle_of_motivation.

31 Gallup, 'Item 3: Doing What I Do Best', Gallup, 5 April 1999, https://www.gallup.com/workplace/237542/item-doing-best.aspx.

Serene

Actually, I will argue this with you. You can look it up yourself, but one of the drivers of early childhood development is mastery.[32] The only reason we've been able to walk is that every time we fall, we are almost compelled to try again and again. And if you look at a young child doing anything at all that is non-academically related, you will find this to be true. When they fail to do something, they will try again and again until they've succeeded. And even after they've succeeded, they will still try again and again until they've mastered the task. This is a very innate human drive that unfortunately is damaged by schooling and by work. Because when you bring extrinsic motivators into the equation, you damage the intrinsic motivators. I remember a study stating that more extrinsic motivation actually lowers intrinsic motivation.[33] And the intrinsic motivation in most humans is mastery. I'm not sure if you are a computer gamer, but I am, and you will find that computer gamers spend an inordinate amount of time doing stuff like getting rid of low-level enemies again and again just to be able to gain mastery and go up into the next level. The whole computer gaming industry is based on this need for achievement and this need for mastery. Without this innate human need, the whole computer game industry will just collapse. I will tell you from being a gamer—most gaming is not fun. Killing 500 low-level mushrooms just to go from level two to level three is not fun. But it is innate. And mastery is the second factor for happiness at work.

The third one is social connections. Being with people whom you enjoy, you respect, and whom you trust. Google introduced

---

[32] Edward L. Deci, and Richard M. Ryan, 'Self-determination theory', *Handbook of Theories of Social Psychology* 1, (2012): 416–436, https://doi.org/10.4135/9781446249215.n21.

[33] Dragana Jovanovic and Marina Matejevic, 'Relationship between Rewards and Intrinsic Motivation for Learning - Researches Review', *Procedia - Social and Behavioral Sciences* 149, 5 (2014): 456–460, https://doi.org/10.1016/j.sbspro.2014.08.287.

this new term, psychological safety.[34] I think the better word is trust. The author Stephen Covey wrote about this in *The Speed of Trust*.[35]

MK

Yes, I read that, a long time ago.

Serene

So basically, it's trust. And Dan Pink's talk[36] explains that these are the three things that make people truly love and thrive in what they do.

Then we get back to self-love. I will say that work doesn't teach people self-love. I'm in several mothers' groups, and I observed that our lack of self-love can cast this shadow on our children. I will give you a very simple example. There is a mother who is constantly struggling with her child's math homework. She basically said that she is terrified of math. She said, 'As a mother, I'm terrified of math too. I am terrified that my child will struggle with math the way that I have my entire life. And therefore, when I look at my child, I feel the need to pressurize her to improve her math.'

Then I asked her, 'Could it be that the reason the child is not doing well in math is because the child can feel that you are terrified of math?' Because every time the conversation is about anything to do with math, this mother will say, 'You ladies are so good at it, I'm so lousy at it, I'm so bad at math.' I told her, 'If you constantly say this, your child is going to get this impression

---

[34] Alexander Newman, Ross Donohue and Nathan Eva, 'Psychological safety: A systematic review of the literature', *Human Resource Management Review* 27, 3 (2017): 521–535, https://doi.org/10.1016/j.hrmr.2017.01.001.

[35] Stephen Covey, *The Speed of Trust*, 1st ed. (New York: Free Press, 2006).

[36] Pink, 'The puzzle of motivation'.

that *oh my goodness, even my mum cannot deal with this, so this must be a real terrible thing, right? Even my mum, who is so capable, has problems with math.*' And she's a very successful businesswoman who basically runs the household and the business. What does that tell you about math? When we talk about self-love, this is what I mean. The shadows that we cast.

I don't know whether you've heard of this term, *use of self.* It's an organizational development term, but also picked up a lot by consultants, and it means *we don't bring our baggage to the company.* We, as consultants and leaders, need to have cleared our personal traumas and shadows to the extent that we are clean instruments. When we walk into a company, we are not projecting our own insecurities, traumas and baggage on to the situation and on to the company. Because only then can we truly see the problem for what it is and solve it. I will tell you this: it's easy to do this as a consultant, but it's extremely hard to do this as a parent. I will say, in terms of level of difficulty, being a clean instrument for the consultancy is not such a big challenge, but to be a clean instrument as a parent, oh my goodness, it's like a whole different level of mastery altogether.

MK

Yep.

Serene

And we constantly project on to our children. When you're talking about self-love, this is what I think about. And if you look at it in terms of a mental health situation, then a lot of what we project out into the world is really our baggage, right? I mean, just look at the differing responses to everything, from COVID to work from home. Earlier on, you mentioned how everybody wants to stay at home. I know a lot of people, including myself, by the way, who would love nothing more than to go back to the office. So, what is the response that you have? Similarly, on the other side, as the manager, what is the response to people going 'I want to stay at home'? If your response is, *'No, how can you stay at home? You'll not get any work done,' is* that a projection of the manager's insecurity, or a read of the actual situation?

MK

Then we're looking at a performance index. If we can still work no matter where we're at, then it shouldn't be a problem.

Serene

Look, regarding the whole 'working from home is not an entitlement', 'companies are not obliged to allow you to work from home' and so on situation, I will tell you honestly: it's a projection rather than an evaluation. Whenever I see that, I see it as a reflection of self-love. I agree with you that it should be based on a performance index. Unfortunately, most work and business decisions are not made based on that. A lot of the decisions are made based more on who I am, than what is happening. And the more threatening a situation is, the more people default to their most comfortable way of operating, which usually means that that is their prejudices and stereotypes talking. Which is why there are all these BLM[37] movements and #MeToo[38] movements going on, and all that. Because the more threatening a situation, the more bigotry and prejudice are shown.

MK

But I feel all these interventions, even if we do it from the outside, it's still an external intervention, whereas internal interventions

[37] BLM: Black Lives Matter, a sociopolitical movement protesting against incidents of police brutality and all racially motivated violence against black people.

[38] #MeToo: A social movement against sexual abuse and sexual harassment where people publicize allegations of sex crimes.

still lie in the level of awareness and ownership that the person has towards themself and towards what they choose to apply their energies and consciousness to.

CULTIVATING PSYCHOLOGICAL SAFETY IN THE WORKPLACE

MK

So how can people gain clarity, to recognize that there is a spillover on their personal end into the team and organizational interest and goals?

Serene

There are two ways about this. Obviously, an individual can do self-work and gain greater self-awareness and understanding of the projections that they're coming from, that's one way. The other direction is this . . . I'll give you an example. I'm sure you belong to a family where there are different family members, and very likely these family members all bring their baggage to the family unit and project on each other. Many times, this causes unhappiness, but I am also going on another presumption, which is that you have a basically functioning family unit: you're not being threatened with your life every day and people are not walking out all the time. What causes this basic family unit to still function despite all the projections that we bring to it? And as I told you earlier on, as a parent, I find it extremely difficult not to project. If you ask me, it goes back to the same quality that we talked about earlier on, which Google identified in their research as the number one most important for team performance—psychological safety. When you are at home, you feel psychologically safe. You trust that your family members are looking out for you, are not actively out to kill you, and the family members trust you the same way. And that is the premise required for a family to work.

The moment you lose that, that's it. In a team, I'm not saying we're all going to be one big happy family, please don't—

MK

Are we talking about safe spaces?

Serene

Okay, my definition of psychological safety is that it's the basic trust that I can be real and vulnerable with you, and you will not seek to make use of that information to harm me. That is the basic trust. It doesn't mean we agree with each other or even that we like each other. But the basic trust is that even when I'm real and vulnerable with you, you're not going to hurt me. And in a team, that is core. I will say this. If your premise of teamwork is a group of enlightened individuals who all come with great self-awareness and do not bring their projections into the team, good luck! The truth is people all come with their baggage. We spend more time with our colleagues than we spend at home and all that baggage, all that projection, is going to come up, especially when we're under stress, especially when there's a deadline due, especially when I've got to see you day in day out. So, what then causes the team to still be able to function? It's very simple. The fact that I trust that, even if I have behaved badly today, tomorrow I can still go to you and apologize for it.

MK

And I can still correct the error.

Serene

And we will still be able to work. So that's the basic trust. When you look at workplace mental health, this sense of psychological safety is extremely important, and it's important on two levels.

On an organizational level, that is what we call the culture. Many Fortune 500 companies actively encourage internal competition. Staff fight to kill one another. In that kind of environment, would you ever feel safe? That's one issue.

The second half of it is this. I think there's almost an acknowledgement, in this time, of a shared sense of catastrophe. Because there's a lot happening worldwide. In Singapore, we are quite fortunate. But in the workplace, there may be people who come from India. For example, I just had a colleague break down and cry to me because of what's happening back home in her country in India. And what about places like Europe? I've had colleagues share about this prevalent sense of *I don't know what's going to happen next* that their families are feeling. When their families cry to them, how would they feel? They can't leave, they can't go there, can't even drop by for a visit, can't even take two weeks off for a holiday and go there to help their families out any more. People are facing real crises, and this is no joke. What do you do as a leader, what do you do as a team? Are you there to say, *Sorry, this is your portion of your work, please get it done and let us know when you're done.*

Then, let's look at our work environment now and the reasons why I yearn to go back to the office. One of the things that we've taken out of Zoom calls is we've taken out the social interaction. Previously in the office, we sat next to each other, so throughout the day I could maybe crack jokes with you. We could go out for coffee. We can have a meeting, and everybody will take a cup of coffee, sit there, and spend probably ten minutes grousing about this and that before we start our meeting. Or we go to the water cooler. We have lunch together. There are all of these social interactions that we don't do on a Zoom call. We have back-to-back Zoom calls and the moment you get on, it is business, set, done, one hour, next Zoom call, next Zoom call, next Zoom call. And it's isolating. You lose the ability to take a break.

Thirdly, you lose the social bonding and social support network is one of the big components of resilience according to research.[39] Your resilience is dependent on how many people you have behind you supporting you. This was shared with me by a psychiatrist, through some research where he found that the strength of your resilience is really the strength of your social support network. And when that social gel goes, no one on earth is mentally strong enough. There's no such thing.

In terms of workplace health, I would say two things for individuals. We need, A, to know that we're not superhumans. I've lost track of the number of times I've told people in these past one and a half years, *you are not superhuman, take a break. No job is worth your life.* That's the other one I've been saying. You're human, so plan your meetings for forty-five minutes or fifty minutes, then take a break. Go to the kitchen, take a drink, like what you would do in the office. Do two minutes of stretching, play with your dog, play with your cat, whatever. Then come back to work again. Secondly, schedule Zoom calls specifically to connect to people. This is the job of the leader. Once a week minimum, schedule a Zoom call that just says we're just going to come on, we're just going to check in with each other, see what's happening with everybody this week. Even if you have to cut down the time that you spend on actual work, cut down! Because nobody's going to be working if they're mentally stressed out and dying, right? You've heard of distress and eustress, haven't you?

MK

Yeah.

Serene

At a certain level of stress, your mind goes into tunnel vision, and you stop being able to think creatively, connect to people, and you

[39] Faith Ozbay et al., 'Social Support and Resilience to Stress', *Psychiatry* (Edgmont) 4, 5 (2007), 35–40, https://www.ncbi.nlm.nih.gov/pmc/articles/PMC2921311/.

stop being able to process, right? What happens when people are stressed out is they're not doing their best work, and they make more mistakes, or make—

MK

They make more errors even if the error is something they shouldn't have made.

Serene

Correct. They make more errors, they have more tunnel vision. This is all information on the human psychology.[40] So these days, you have a group of people who are all under stress, right? Now, if it's just within Singapore, it's not so bad. I think probably the CB[41] period was the worst, but now we've kind of settled down a bit. But there are still people who are looking at their family members in other countries that are being affected. They have friends in other countries that are being affected. The other thing that's happening is people are worried about this year. Because last year, we had a ton of money that the government pumped into the system. But will this year mean more retrenchment? People are worried and concerned about the instability.

And Singapore is so small! We're so outwardly dependent. How long can our economy sustain this? We cannot sustain it internally, we know this for a fact. People have very real concerns and to just go like *let's do business as usual*—it's too unrealistic and too unproductive.

MK

It's like saying let's forget about everything that's happening in this world and just do our work.

---

[40] Habib Yaribeygi et al, 'The Impact of Stress on Body Function: A Review', *EXCLI Journal* 16, (2017), 1057–1072, doi: 10.17179/excli2017-480.

[41] CB: Circuit Breaker refers to the three month nationwide lockdown in Singapore to curb the spread of COVID-19.

Serene

Yes, but it's very unproductive, right? Because how many humans do you know are able to completely cut off their emotional state and focus?

MK

We can't. Most people can't.

Serene

I'm sure you can if you're like the Dalai Lama or somebody, but most people can't, right?

MK

That's why they bring in all their projections and baggage into the workplace as well. It's a spillover.

Serene

It's fine. Look, it just means you are human. And as humans, I think most colleagues do care for each other. Just sit there and go, *Hey, how have things been with you?* Like the same question you asked me today, *are you all right?* And to have a genuine response like *I'm not very all right* and have that real conversation, even if it's ten minutes a day. I think that's very, very helpful and what people need at the moment. So, two things are, one, take breaks; two, have social connection.

THE SHOES OF A LEADER

Serene

There is a third thing, and it's for the leader. And I will say this is in contradiction to the previous point, and therefore, to be frank, it's a little bit hard to expect leaders to do, because the next one is you need to project confidence.

MK

That's the job of the leader—to give everybody the confidence and clear vision of what we're moving towards.

Serene

Correct. But the thing is, right now, most leaders do not have a clear vision themselves. And secondly, we talked about how leaders should be authentic and vulnerable. And being authentic and vulnerable means that the leader is probably also feeling anxious, is also feeling stressed out, right? So as a leader, where do you draw the line between how real you need to be and how confident you need to be?

MK

Appropriateness.

Serene

To be frank, the challenge of the leader . . . you need to consider a few things. The first is the maturity of the team members. I mean, the more mature they are, obviously the more real you can be. If you're leading a bunch of very young people, then you need to be more confident. The second one is the emotional connection between everybody, right? If you're in a team that has really gelled together, worked together for a while, everybody knows everybody very well and we are very familiar with each other, then you can be more real. If it's a newer team that's just gotten together, especially if you've got people recruited since last year and you haven't even seen them since last year or you haven't even seen them in real life, then you might need to project a bit more confidence. And the third one is, as you probably can imagine, the nature of the job. In more critical, time-stressed jobs, you need to be more confident. If it's a bit more of a creative job, then you might need to be more authentic because people need to be more creative, more relaxed. So where do you really draw the line as a leader?

MK

It's a tough job.

Serene

Well, you know, that's why they get paid well! Every time they complain to me, I'll say, 'No, that's why you get paid more. You have more prestige, you have more power! What are you complaining about?' Sorry, I'm not very sympathetic. But that is the truth that leaders are facing at the moment. Another struggle that leaders are facing right now is, *what do I do about team members that are not performing due to mental health issues?*

MK

Yeah.

Serene

I've lost track of the number of leaders who've come to me saying, 'I've this team member. They've always been working very well, but since last year, they have just not been working. They're missing deadlines, not doing their jobs. When I talk to them, they don't seem to know what's happening.' That kind of thing. Then the question that follows is, *Do you think they need a counsellor?* What do you do with these people? Do you say, *You're not performing, therefore I need to move you off the team, counsel you to leave?* Do you say, *You're not performing, therefore I ask you to see a counsellor?* Is that appropriate? Will MOM[42] come after me if I tell you, *Buddy, I think you're struggling, perhaps you need to go*

[42] MOM: Ministry of Manpower

and see a counsellor? Are leaders allowed to say that to their people? And I always tell them to be careful about what they say, because you are not allowed to discriminate against people due to mental health conditions. And the very act of saying, *I think you should see a psychiatrist,* can be misconstrued as discrimination, especially if after that, you are forced to let them go.

MK

Yeah. And employees can use that to go against them.

Serene

Correct. Then what do you do as a leader? How do you say it as a leader? These are all things that leaders are struggling with right now—real issues, not funny at all. Like, I have this person, and normally they perform quite well, but ever since COVID, they have not been performing. It's been a year, what do I do? I've done all the performance counselling and coaching that I know how to do as a leader, I've told them *Hey, you're not performing up to standard, you need to do better.* I've given clearer instructions, better delegation, gone to talk to them. What do I do now? Do I fire them? I have all the track records of them not performing for a year and a half. I can if I want to. But is it fair? To fire somebody who does perform, can perform, but suddenly seems to be having a mental health issue?

MK

I'm stuck now. If I'm in that position, I realize that I don't know what to do.

Serene

Yeah, and I'm sure there are cold-hearted people out there who are like, *just get rid of them*, but for the leaders that are genuine, they care for their people. They are real as human beings. They know what these people are facing, and I don't think that they are the sort of people that just cut them off.

MK

I'm getting confronted by this conversation. Heavy stuff. Because every choice that you make does have a huge impact on the other person.

Serene

Yes, correct. And I will throw in another can of worms, which is that you're not just responsible for this one person. You may have six people on your team. One is not performing, which means the other five people are pulling the additional work. Are you being fair to the five people if you say, *I think this person has a mental health issue, would you let them hang on?* There are more implications as a leader. It sets a very bad example, a very bad precedent. I mean, I don't have the answers. I will not say I have the answers for these. But when you talk about workplace mental health, I will say that these are the challenges that real people struggle with. And workplace mental health is becoming more and more of an issue. Maybe some are non-performing. The rest of them are still performing. So, let's say 60 per cent are more anxious, and have a 10 per cent to 15 per cent drop in their work performance. What's the impact on the organization and the team? They are not performing well, and you are in a situation where you need people to think of new strategies, new ideas, to adapt to this new market, and to try and get better ideas, do better, but we're not bringing our best selves to work. I mean, I certainly will not be if I'm anxious, right? Obviously, I think this anxiety could be a whole spectrum. There could be people way down on the anxiety scale who are calm. And maybe some people are only 3 per cent to 5 per cent different. But let's say I give you an average of 15 per cent difference? Is that a lot? Probably.

MK

That's quite a lot!

Serene

And you multiply that by more than half the organization. There are lots of statistics, you know.[43] There's a lot of unprocessed grief in the world at the moment.[44] The empathetic people who are usually the social gel of any team are the most affected, because when they look at the world, they look at how people are suffering. Therefore, they have a harder time coping, and these are the very people who gel the team together. They're what I call social lubricants: they make everything go well. When these people are not coping, imagine the team dynamics. If you are the social gel and you're not functioning as well, what happens to the team dynamics? Nobody is actively working, so all the hard drivers, taskmasters, will dominate, right? There's all this stuff that's happening on a team and organizational level and people don't think it's important at all. One of the reasons why I'm doing a weekly show about this is because I want people to know it's happening! It's real!

MK

To be honest, I didn't really know what you really do with organizations until today.

Serene

Then how did you get hold of me?

---

[43] Gabriele Giorgi et al., 'COVID-19-Related Mental Health Effects in the Workplace: A Narrative Review', *Int J Environ Res Public Health* 17, 21 (2020), 7857, https://pubmed.ncbi.nlm.nih.gov/33120930/.

[44] Maarten C. Eisma, Paul A. Boelen and Lonneke I.M. Lenferink, 'Prolonged grief disorder following the Coronavirus (COVID-19) pandemic', *Psychiatry Res* 288, 113031 (2020), https://doi.org/10.1016/j.psychres.2020.113031.

MK

I know that you're a performance coach, but I didn't know the extent of what you do with corporates in the organization. I always thought you worked with individuals, groups, organizations, but I didn't have the knowledge that you actually work with the other side first. Because that means the loop is actually complete. Your perspective and understanding of how the whole thing works is complex.

Serene

That's why when I was talking to you, I kept pushing you.

MK

You were pushing me, you know, and, *wow*, this was one of the hardest conversations I've had.

[Serene laughs]

CHAPTER 5

Scaffolding Layers of Support for Mental Health

By Tin Pei Ling, Member of Parliament,
MacPherson SMC

In the community, mental health usually comes to the fore when the more serious types of mental health issues precipitate into other types of behavioural issues. Tin Pei Ling shares some of the community tensions that were caused by persons with mental health conditions, and the challenges faced by neighbours living with these tensions daily.

HOW MENTAL HEALTH PRECIPITATES INTO OTHER ISSUES

MK

In your position as a leader working with the community and people on the ground, what are some of the mental health issues that you've observed are happening?

Tin Pei Ling

I think the term 'mental health issues' is quite broad. In popular media, mental health issues are usually typecast as being serious, requiring medical attention, and may include commonly reported types such as depression, psychosis, and OCD.[45] OCD is not psychosis, of course, but these are the issues we often hear about in the media.

But there are other instances of mental health struggles that may not be so obvious to people, and should perhaps be seen as part of a broader concept of 'mental wellness' as emotions and moods lie on a spectrum and can be triggered by the immediate environment. For example, in recent times, it has been very stressful for many people and that stress, worry, etc., can lead to anxieties and even exacerbate some of the anti-social behaviour that we observe in people around us. It's like how we talk about general health. Mental health can also cover quite a broad range when we talk about it.

Within the community, mental health usually comes to the fore when the more serious types of mental health issues precipitate into other types of behavioural issues. Take, for example, a couple of years ago, there was a case of very frequent high-rise littering. The neighbour on the ground floor had to bear the brunt of it because the rubbish landed in front of the door and he and

[45] OCD: Obsessive Compulsive Disorder

his family had to face it every time they opened the door. Upon investigation, we managed to identify the unit and the person who did was a neighbour with a mental health issue who had an IMH[46] record. When explaining to the affected neighbour, the neighbour made a comment I thought was worth further deliberation. The affected neighbour said, 'While I understand and empathize, this is happening to us on a daily basis'. Essentially, if such incidents happen once in a while, perhaps they may tolerate it. But when it happens every day and they have to bear with the consequences, they will find it hard to accept. Therefore, I'm afraid that that adds to the stigma. Hence, when we address mental health issues, we have to address them from different angles. What I have just shared is an illustration of some of the complex challenges faced in addressing mental health in the community.

Adding another layer is our ageing population. With ageing more people are expected to have Alzheimer's or dementia. Many people see this as part of mental health too. MacPherson is a mature estate and we have more seniors. So, what can we do to help seniors with dementia and their caregivers so that they can have a better quality of life? At home, I think that's something we cannot freely intervene in. But within the community, what can we do to help them? For instance, MacPherson is a dementia-friendly community (DFC) and it has been so for a while. It's an ongoing journey and we'll continue exploring how we can strengthen it. Part of being a DFC is about having dementia-friendly focal points. These are places where people may naturally gather, where these seniors may naturally go to, and what we do is to equip the people who hang around there could be hawkers, could be shopkeepers, could be neighbours–with the knowledge and ability to identify signs of dementia. If you see someone looking lost, how do you step forward to help? How do you ask them and determine whether this is a person with dementia who

[46] IMH: Institute of Mental Health

is lost? What can we do to help this senior find his or her way back to their loved ones? These seniors usually have routines. How can we make that routine safer for them so that they can go out, enjoy their day, then go home safely? These are some examples.

Rounding back to what I mentioned earlier, when we talk about mental health issues, we have to look at them from a holistic point of view. Sometimes you cannot look at it from purely a 'health' aspect. There's also a social element. In MacPherson, we created a taskforce a couple of years ago. This is a network of community partners comprising the grassroots, local voluntary welfare organizations and various government agencies. These partners come together to discuss cases and explore how they can collaborate to address the issues from a multidisciplinary case management approach. For example, IMH or SAMH[47] will address the mental health element to either convince the person to seek professional help, because we cannot force them, or if the person has medicine prescribed, to help them adhere to their medication regime. Then, the SSO[48] or the VWO[49] will step in to offer financial or employment assistance, so that the person can focus on recovery or regaining normalcy in life. Of course, different cases have different circumstances, and different solutions are required. But basically, taking a holistic approach to cases is essential.

ON STIGMA: REALITY LIES IN THE PERCEPTION OF OTHERS

MK

Got it. What are some stigmas you have observed as you are on the ground?

---

[47] SAMH: Singapore Association of Mental Health

[48] SSO: Social Service Office

[49] VWO: Voluntary Welfare Organisation

Tin Pei Ling

Some people may still misunderstand mental health as just psychosis. There is nothing wrong with psychosis, per se, but past perceptions, or how mental health is portrayed in dramas and thriller movies, may have instilled fear, leading to discriminatory behaviours—knowingly or unknowingly. These add to the stigma. Some people with a mood disorder or depression may find themselves unwilling to seek help as they fear being labelled by others, 人言可畏[50], which is very stressful.

MK

What do you think is holding people back from seeking help, especially when they are aware that they're going through certain difficulties in life where they need to look for support systems, but yet, they are still not able to step forward?

Tin Pei Ling

I think it has to go back to stigma. If you think about it, if I have the flu, I have no qualms about going to the doctor and getting an MC.[51] But when it comes to mental health, people are a lot more reserved about it. Of course, it could also be due to awareness. Sometimes, people don't know when to seek help. *Is this sadness that I'm feeling just a passing phase? Or am I just useless or weak?* Sometimes they have self-defeating thoughts, and they think, *Maybe it's just one of those phases.* They don't seek help, they don't pay attention to it, but then it gets worse after a while. But as I mentioned, there's also the stigma. If you realize that you need help but are not seeking it, what is stopping you? Is it because you're afraid of people looking at you differently? Looking down on you or shunning you? Et cetera, et cetera. This can be terrifying because

---

[50] 人言可畏: Mandarin phrase meaning 'words can be hurtful'

[51] MC: Medical Certificate.

humans are social beings, and nobody likes to be discriminated or 被人家白眼.[52]

Other factors preventing people who need help from getting help could include whether the caregiver or family knows about the condition, whether the family members have the capacity and time to talk to them, or take them to seek professional help.

MK

I'm aware that you work with the youth, elderly, and young families. I'm wondering, do the mental health stigmas vary between these different groups?

Tin Pei Ling

I think the root cause, or the underlying factor, is similar: stigma is a huge issue.

One difference is that the degree of awareness varies between generations. The understanding of what constitutes mental health in the older generation will differ from the younger folks because there's so much being talked about today. Mental health today, versus just a few years ago, is in a very different state. For instance, the tone and volume of responses I get for my social media posts on mental health today are much better than similar posts from years ago.

Of course, finances are a contributing factor too. If one gets diagnosed with a mental health condition, it is not as if 今天吃药, 明天好[53], right? It may last for a while, and one will then think of how to afford it over the longer term. This could be a cause for worry for some.

---

[52] 被人家白眼: Mandarin phrase meaning 'be looked down upon'

[53] 今天吃药, 明天好: Mandarin phrase meaning 'you will immediately get better after a dose of medication'

WE NEED TO BE EXPLICIT IN EXPRESSING SUPPORT

MK

Thank you for that. Is there anything else you would like to add?

Tin Pei Ling

Well, I do think that we're in a better position today.

MK

Consider our recent times. Even though COVID has triggered a lot of stress, there is greater recognition of the impact of mental health and the need to address it. Many people are very stressed, and we see it being manifested in different ways—having shorter tempers, and sometimes it could even precipitate into behaviours that they would never have thought, under normal circumstances, could happen. For example, Asian hate, right? These are things that are worrying. But in general, people are more open to talking about mental health today. People recognize that this is nothing to be ashamed of. This is just part of our health, everyone is different, and we should look into addressing it. Simply put, if we don't help people with mental wellness, their potential can be curtailed. What do I mean? If an individual is struggling with his internal battles, it takes attention, takes energy away from his school, his career, his family. And that would be a shame. That would be a pity. So, if we can support them in addressing those battles so that they can better focus on what really matters to them, I think we can see a lot more potential being fulfilled, and that would be wonderful.

And the situation is better today. From the proxy indicator I get . . . last time when I talked about mental health on social media, the number of likes or responses I got compared to other posts were very low. Whereas last year and this year, I realized that there's a lot more expressed support, and I think it's a good sign that we should continue on that momentum.

MK

How do you think, as a community, we can move forward more powerfully together to tackle mental health issues?

Tin Pei Ling

I think a lot has been said about awareness, about tolerance, about understanding. These are all true, but it doesn't happen overnight. I think there are a few things. Firstly, everyone has to be more explicit in their support. If people can be more open about expressing their support, their willingness to work with each other, I think that's useful. The community of support is also important. For example, earlier on I talked about how MacPherson works with different agencies and organizations to see how we can, in a more holistic manner, help individuals with their mental health needs. I think that the support and scaffold need to be there. In the end, it's still a journey. People need to understand that it's a process. I don't think we are fully *fully* there yet, but I think it's a lot better now.

APPROACHING MENTAL HEALTH RESPONSIBLY

MK

One of the things in my space is this. With more awareness, it also creates a new problem. Every time a person feels stressed, they tend to associate themselves with certain factors and self-diagnose themselves without having seen a professional, just based on a few online articles and social media posts that they read. How do you think we can counter that? To make sure that information doesn't become misinformation, because it is inevitable in the digital space.

Tin Pei Ling

I think it's about knowing what mental health is, what the different conditions are, and what the spectrum of symptoms is. Just as you would understand what's cancer, what's flu, what's gastroenteritis, etc., the same goes for mental health. When everyone takes mental health seriously and in the right spirit, we can address biases, avoid irresponsible excuses, and make positive progress.

MK

I think it goes back to the equation of how we can fundamentally be more responsible as individuals, how we can also develop a sense of ontological humility, rather than take advantage of stuff like this, that may actually worsen the existing stigmas around mental health.

Tin Pei Ling

I agree. I think we just need to be mindful.

CHAPTER 6

No One Is Exempt from Mental Health Challenges

By Seah Kian Peng, Member of Parliament, Chairperson of Braddel Heights (Marine Parade GRC)

In our circle of family and friends, we probably know someone who has gone through mental health challenges. For Seah Kian Peng, it was a primary schoolmate who lost his son to suicide. As a community leader, Seah Kian Peng shares that it is important to create safe spaces for people to engage or consult a mental health professional. Many people worry that they would be seen in a different light if they shared their struggles. As such, he highlights the importance of both awareness and acceptance in society in order for people to feel safe enough to reach out for help.

THE STRESSES PEOPLE FACE ARE MORE FREQUENT AND COMPLEX

Seah Kian Peng

Over the years, many of us, both inside and outside Parliament, have raised the issue of mental health. I have raised this topic in some of my speeches. And at the practical level, I have worked with Silver Ribbon to set up a centre in my constituency. For me, what is critical is to create more awareness around this topic as it is very real and important. No stigma should be attached to it. If you ask me, I think every one of us, whoever you are, is likely to experience some of these challenges at some point in time—as a young person, as a student, as an adult, as a teenager, whatever. We will all have these moments. Therefore, coming to terms with it and knowing how to deal with it is very important. In fact, I'm sure we know of friends or family members who have gone through mental health challenges. Some come out of it, some unfortunately succumb to it, and some are continuing to deal with it.

And actually, not so long ago, one of my primary schoolmates shared with us that . . . actually, the funeral was last week. His son . . . I think he was in the UK . . . my schoolmate wasn't aware that his son was dealing with depression, and unfortunately, he took his life. It's very sad. And there are many of these examples. This is why I support the mental health cause, because I think every one of us, *every one of us*, needs to know about it. I would say that most of us know how to deal with it. There are those of us who discover some coping strategies along the way, but unfortunately, there's also quite a big group who don't know how to deal with their mental health challenges and, as a result, cause a lot of grief and harm to themselves and the people around them. It is good that you all are doing this. It's something I'm totally supportive of. And the more people know about it, the better the community will be.

MK

Got it.

Because you're a leader working with the community, whether it is with people on the ground, or people in leadership positions, what are the mental health stigmas you've observed in Singapore?

Seah Kian Peng

Firstly, I have noticed that when a person says that they have a mental health issue, immediately the image that is cast on the person changes. Some may wonder if there's something about this person that they should distance themselves from, or whether it reflects what their family is like. I think this shouldn't be the case. That's why awareness is important.

Actually, perhaps what's more important is the environment—whether it's family, friends, or the workplace. It's more important that the stakeholders in those spaces respond to these things, either to call it out, and then find ways to work with the person to help them get out of this, or to seek treatment. If I use the workplace as an example, maybe more so now than before, stress is something that we all have to deal with, and COVID has added another layer of stress to a lot of us. At workplaces, certainly at mine, what we've done in this past year was to set up a counselling service. We call it Care Angel, and anyone who's facing issues can just reach out, obviously with confidentiality and anonymity guaranteed. It is so they know there's a place, a safe space, a number to call, a person to see or talk to, to help them tide through challenging periods. If you have such services, that will help at the community level. At the constituency level, I know it's important to have that too, which is why when Silver Ribbon came to us wanting to set up a centre to provide mental wellness services, we said, *Sure, let's set it up.*

What I'm getting at is number one, we need to create as many of these safe spaces for people to be able to engage or consult a mental health professional when needed at the workplace or in the residential areas. The other aspect is raising the general awareness that mental health is something which all of us—and I'm repeating what I said earlier—will go through. Hand to heart, ask yourself: *Have you had those moments where you had a lot on your mind, many thoughts going on at the same time? How did you deal with it?* It is normal to have these experiences. Some may be real. Some may be perceived. Some may be self-created, self-doubts you impose on yourself. Some are certainly caused by the environment. The part about raising the general awareness and understanding and destigmatizing these things is one important area. Once you have that, the next step is to create safe spaces for people to get help. And to let them know that it is okay to get help. In fact, there are things you must get help for and not try to solve by yourself, because some things are not so straightforward.

I think you need to have both. If you ask me now, compared to ten years ago, even five years ago, are we in a better space as a whole? I think so. But it doesn't change the fact that the world is getting more complicated. The stresses that everyone faces have also intensified and become more frequent and complex as well. While the facilities, the infrastructure, the general awareness and understanding have improved, unfortunately, the stresses and issues that every single individual faces are on a different level, which is why you see more of such cases coming up. Maybe there were already some of these cases, but it was a case of underreporting that disguised or masked the actual number. Perhaps the lines of communication, like social media, have brought to light many of these things, but it may not necessarily reflect that the situation is worse than before. Just some of my thoughts.

GIVING VOICE TO WHAT'S UNSAID

MK

A lot of people attribute COVID or the lockdown as the factors that caused mental health issues, emotional wellness issues, and others. I disagree with that to a certain extent. I think COVID is an event that accentuated and surfaced a lot of things that we have buried inside us. Considering that we live a very fast-paced life, sometimes we don't even have the opportunity to slow down, look inside ourselves, and notice that something's off. And oftentimes, I think many of us actually brush it aside as a coping mechanism.

Seah Kian Peng

Ming Kwang, I agree with you on that. Because of COVID, we are staying home more, and we interact with our family members more. And I think through that, certain issues become more apparent. Because you're interacting more, you're spending more time with each other, you actually see those issues more. They may have already been there, but because your interactions were not as frequent, perhaps they were hidden deep inside. But now, these issues have surfaced and become more obvious.

MK

Correct. Which means more opportunities for us as individuals to work on those issues, because we can't spend our time running away from it.

Seah Kian Peng

True. Which is why I think the more we talk about it, it will certainly help. I'm obviously not an expert on this, but I think talking about anything is always better than not talking about it. Sometimes we just need time to air our issues out, and after we air them out, we feel better. And that, for some, may be all that's needed.

MK

You're saying that it's about saying the unsaid?

Seah Kian Peng

Saying the unsaid, number one, and knowing that the unsaid is something that is not peculiar to you. If you ask me, have I gone through some of these episodes? *Sure.* I think when I was a student, at different points in time in my life journey, different issues surfaced. Now when I look back, would those be classified as moments where it's a mental health issue? These are things you battled inside your head, inside yourself: are these classified as mental health issues? *Probably.* In that definition, did I also have those moments? *Yes*, as I'm sure many others would have too. Maybe everyone would have them at some point in their life. For those who have it really bad, I want to tell them, *it's okay.* You're not alone.

I think the key message is that you are not alone. For some people who feel that they're alone, that *I have to deal with it alone, I'm the odd one out*, that sometimes leads to unfortunate consequences. And that's what we hope to prevent because many of these things can be treated and can be overcome. And while it might be tough, just talking about it and receiving treatment versus not treating it. The outcomes are quite different.

MK

I think there's also a saying that if we want to help other people, we have to help ourselves first.

Seah Kian Peng

Totally. For example, as you know, I'm at FairPrice. I always say first we have to take care of our staff, but to take care of your staff, you got to take care of yourself first. If you can't take care of yourself, how can you take care of your staff and look after your customers? I totally agree with you that it starts with me first. And the more I know about it, the more I know how to seek help, then first I can help myself, and then in turn I can help others. And there's nothing more powerful than someone who has gone through it, dealt with it, and is now able to tell others about it.

IT'S AN EVERYDAY CONVERSATION, NOT AN OVERNIGHT FIX

MK

What do you think is holding individuals back from seeking help? Let's say a person is going through certain mental health challenges. There needs to be a willingness in them to want to ask for help and engage in these resources already available in Singapore.

Seah Kian Peng

I'll go back to the earlier point when you talked about the unsaid. The perception is, *If I have this, what would others think about me? What would my family think about me? What would my friends think about this? Would I be accepted in the community, in the groups that I interact with?* I think, to me, that is the biggest barrier. And probably that causes a lot of unnecessary stress. And therefore, if you turn this whole thing around, one part is about 'me', but the other part is the 'people around me'. Family, friends, colleagues, neighbours, whatever—I think that is probably very, *very* stressful! All these probably even overpower everything else.

Even if I accept myself, I then have to look at the other side of things which is how the rest of the community, the people, look at me. Even if I can deal with it myself, the rest of the people may not accept me. I have to battle with myself first, then I have to battle with the rest. I think we need both—acceptance and awareness in the self and in the community. It's not mutually exclusive. It's not binary. You need both to work, and both to help each other.

MK

How does knowing all of this shape your approach as a leader?

Seah Kian Peng

First is raising awareness, and then setting up support systems. You still need all these support systems, and they must be accessible so that people know where they can get help if they need it. And the third part is sharing. It takes courage to open up, for anyone. If you're able to get people to open up, to share their own personal journeys or experiences, I think that is very powerful because it's very likely that others can better relate to it. Your experiences, my experiences, or our friends' experiences. It will build a sense of realism for these issues, more so if they are spoken by the person who experienced it himself or herself.

I have also organized talks at my CCs[54] to talk about all this. I will chip in with my own views at these talks and get others to do so as well. It's about creating a safe environment for people to talk to and show that it is not a taboo subject. And the more we talk . . . obviously we hope that this is not a one-off thing that we only talk about on World Mental Health Day, but it's—

MK

It's an everyday conversation.

Seah Kian Peng

It's an everyday conversation! It's a conversation we can have across different life stages, right? Kids have exam stress, and

---

[54] CC: Community Centre

parents are stressed too. Then there are boyfriend-girlfriend issues. Work stresses. All kinds of issues. Talk about it, create safe environments, and create the facilities to deal with such things.

I'll use my workplace as an example. We have our counselling service Care Angel, and it is available to anyone who needs help. As the CEO, the only thing I ask them is, '*Has the Care Angel family been used?*' The good news is that it has been used, so I know people actually reach out. I don't know whether it's good or bad news, but the number of people who use it is not a lot lah, which is also not a bad thing. Number one, there aren't so many cases. But number two, it's being used. The worst would outcome would have been that nobody actually called, so it didn't even touch one life. But I know there were a few, and for those who used it, I am quite sure it would have helped him or her. But even if it's one, two, or ten people who use it out of 10,000 people, for those who used it, it mattered to them, it helped them, and so it's worth it. And if you look at the free counselling services Silver Ribbon provides in my constituency, based on the way it's set up, if you don't know what this place is for, if you just look at it from the outside, the centre looks really nice, you know. It creates an atmosphere where people can just walk in comfortably, and that's how it ought to be. Again, I don't think there are many residents who walk in, but are there people who walk in? *Sure.* Whether it's one, ten, or a hundred people who've used it since it opened two years ago, as long as it mattered to them, as long as it made a difference in their lives, that's all we're after.

All these things we do to build a more caring, more inclusive society . . . I think it will always be work in progress. Among other services, we also have a dyslexic learning centre at my constituency at one of the void decks. Having such a centre creates awareness for people who don't know about dyslexia. For some people, this condition creates inconveniences for others, with peers, right? But once you understand it—it doesn't mean the inconveniences will be less—your relationship with your peers gets better because there is that understanding.

But the point I'm getting at is that whether it's dyslexia, whether it's other special needs, whether it's mental health, I think these are things no one should be afraid to talk about. There is nothing to feel bad about. For some, early intervention, early detection, and treatment will help significantly. And in the end, all we're trying to do is tell everyone that every life is precious. We all go through trials and tribulations in different ways. And if there are ways in which, as an individual, as an MP[55] as a CEO, whatever, if there are ways you can play your part to address this, I think we should always take the step forward and not just rely totally on Mr Government. For sure, the government has to play an important role and set up certain agencies to deal with all this, but that alone is not a silver bullet to many things, as we all know.

So likewise, in every estate, there's a SSO[56] in my constituency, and there are also FSCs[57] and such. Overall, I think we need a whole-of-community approach. The religious institutions also come in, and people like yourself as well. Everyone needs to play their part to help make lives better for everyone. These are all very important jobs to be done. And the causes that you're supporting and this book that you're coming up with will certainly take us another step forward in combating stigma and helping us address mental health in a more holistic manner.

---

[55] MP: Member of Parliament

[56] SSO: Social Service Office

[57] FSC: Family Service Center

CHAPTER 7

We Are One Society

By Murali Pillai, Member of Parliament, Bukit Batok SMC

As a police officer and now a Member of Parliament, Murali Pillai witnessed the varied ways mental health manifests in the community. As a community, he believes it is important to create the support structures so that people can access help wherever they're at. To do so, he hopes people can collaborate with openness, as neighbours, mental health professionals and inter-government agencies as well, so that we can support others in a way that best suits them.

MENTAL HEALTH IS A MULTIFACETED ISSUE

Si Qi

What are your thoughts on mental health?

Murali

Well, it's multifaceted, obviously. I would say, my rude introduction to the repercussions of not having a proper programme reaching out to everybody happened in secondary school. One of my schoolmates unfortunately ended his life. I think he was fifteen years old at that time. I still remember my form teacher crying uncontrollably . . . So, that was a rude awakening. Fast forward to when I became a police officer between 1992 and 1995 and then a community leader, I also had to deal with such issues and suicide cases. One that comes to my mind is the case of the father having a heated argument with his boy, who was sixteen years old then. He came back with his school results. His father was so angry with him over the results and told him to *get out of the house.* Unfortunately, the son left the house and ended his life. I spent some time consoling the father, who was so guilt-stricken, and helped him and his wife relocate to another housing estate so that they won't have to replay the incident over and over again in their minds.

Another part of mental health would be in relation to the responsibilities of the caregivers. I've seen a good number of family members bearing the cudgels of responsibility, taking care of their family members who have mental challenges, and it's certainly not easy for them. In my first few years as MP[58] I had the opportunity to talk about this in Parliament and that led to some policy changes. Back then, one only got concessionary

[58] MP: Member of Parliament

levies for migrant domestic workers when one or more family members were physically disabled. I then raised a point, *How about the mentally disabled?* And after a good number of to-ing and fro-ing, the government relented and agreed that families with members who are mentally disabled should also be beneficiaries of this concessionary levy system. Hopefully through this, such families are better assisted.

Later, I set up the Green Ribbon Task Force in Bukit Batok. I started it because there were quite a number of cases involving mentally-challenged persons that were reported to me, more as social disturbances, to be frank—neighbours complaining about other neighbours. The Task Force consists of very committed community leaders who have a little bit of background on mental health issues. They come in to intervene and see whether help can be brought in through our various partners such as hospitals, VWOs[59], and of course committee leaders too. They also help run mental health awareness programmes in the constituency as well. Just to give you another example, there was a complaint about noise being generated in the silent hours, two or three in the morning, by this person who really screams his lungs out. When the Task Force members intervened, it was very clear to them that he had a mental illness. His parents were not very keen to send him for treatment at IMH[60] or some other clinic and would rather get him treated with the traditional religious healers. I highlighted this issue in Parliament and suggested that maybe the mental health professionals could link up with the traditional religious healers, because it's difficult to change the orientation of some residents who truly and fervently believe that such intervention

---

[59] VWO: Voluntary Welfare Organisation

[60] IMH: Institute of Mental Health (Singapore's only hospital dedicated to health health)

can help them or their family members. It's not the best solution, but at least, hopefully, there will be some level of interaction so we can begin to gain some level of confidence and at the end of the day, we can treat this person in a hospital. So, as you can see, it can be very intractable at some level.

And then we realized that caregivers need a lot of support in terms of networks, peer support, knowledge, skill sets. I would like to mention two VWOs in particular, Caregivers Alliance, as well as Care2Care. I think I have attended about seven or eight graduation ceremonies of caregivers who shared very moving testimonies. And so, I heard firsthand how much of a positive impact these classes had on their lives, because they now acquired the skills, they have the knowledge and also formed networks, so they're not alone.

So, you can see, as I'm using the lenses of a community leader and as an MP, it's very clear to me that mental health awareness is not where it should be. We can do a lot more to help people deal with their own mental health issues. We can do a lot more to help caregivers who are supporting these persons and the more partners we have to focus our energies on in this area, the better it would be. We must equip each and every Singaporean with the basic skills to deal with such issues, make them more resilient, make sure they know where to go for help and *never* allow them to feel as though they're helpless.

NETWORK OF NEIGHBOURS HELPING NEIGHBOURS

Si Qi

Thank you for sharing. I think those were very real situations that perhaps not every one of us would have seen.

Murali

I think help is available in Singapore, but there still is an issue of people not wanting to seek help. Through your observations, why do you think there's such a barrier against help-seeking?

We are now in the midst of a pandemic and the government has started the vaccination drive, right? It was suggested that I speak to our seniors about the vaccination and its benefits so that they would sign up, but I realized there is an easier way. I invited our doctor in the neighbourhood who regularly treats our seniors and with whom the seniors have a longstanding relationship over the years. When the doctor said *this is good for you*, it was sealed within minutes!

Murali

Because there's a relationship of trust on the specific issue, you see.

MK

Yeah.

Murali

So there lies the challenge. We may have help and support for our people in these specific areas, but communication is so key and so complex. There are so many factors that determine whether it's at the right level, and getting the right person is important. The Green Ribbon Task Force consists of neighbours and community leaders who are experienced and enjoy the confidence of fellow neighbours. We need to constantly assess and pitch it in an appropriate way so that people really hear the message. Especially now, when there are so many messages.

Again, it takes a network of neighbours helping neighbours. We also have another project called Project Breakthrough where

I have a meeting involving all the different agencies so we can get an updated picture. For each case, there would be various agencies, and I wanted to have a platform where they can share and look at where the gaps are, and I can certainly help to influence some solutions as well. And while the issue may be resolved at one level, it can resurrect itself at another. It's not easy. It's a moving target. We may never be finished with the issue. So as a community, we should also offer a solution. We all have responsibilities. And I think if we say we are one society, we must mean it in our actions.

MK

What made you decide to walk on this path of giving to the community? Because working with people requires a lot of energy and effort. I'm very inspired, that's why I asked that!

Murali

Casting my mind back on my own journey and the help that I've gotten from my mentors, the people who I look up to, I always told myself that if I had an opportunity, I should certainly pay it forward. But when I got myself immersed, I think it was Mahatma Gandhi, who said a long long time ago, 'I best way to find yourself is to lose yourself in the service of others.' Each issue is important. And when you see the issues being tackled, there's a certain sense of calmness from the people who were originally very upset, then you derive a certain satisfaction not because you want to be patted on the back, but you can see that issues are being tackled. Ultimately for me, it's about making sure that our country retains its shape as one community, because I do sincerely believe that that is what is needed to overcome challenges that come our way. That is what is needed to ensure that we continue to enjoy a bright future for every segment of society. It cannot be for the well-off only, it has to be for every segment of society.

COLLABORATION WITH OPENNESS

Si Qi

You were talking about how mental health is a very multifaceted issue, and it's not easy to tackle it from just one angle. What are some of the most urgent gaps that we should be filling up now?

MK

Or tightening?

Murali

We cannot get away from the fact that there is still a stigma associated with mental illness. People of my generation will remember that Woodbridge Hospital is a pejorative phrase. To some extent, it may have driven the behaviour of some families who want to just keep it to themselves despite the fact that help is available. To me, that is an issue that we *must* resolve.

MK

What kind of interventions do you think are necessary?

Murali

We have to normalize mental health issues. Like I said, it's with every one of us.

MK

It involves everybody because we all have a mind, we all have a heart, and we all deal with these difficult emotions.

Murali

Exactly! And every one of us at some point in time would have a mental health issue. It may not be to a level where you need clinical intervention, but we would have those, and we need that scaffolding to help overcome them.

MK

We need to look into that because when we're missing something, we tend to look outwards for answers. But when it comes to looking inwards into ourselves, we don't really have a map. That's why when COVID happened and we were forced to look inwards, domestic violence started increasing. People were forced to deal with family issues that they never really sorted out. Divorce rates actually increased.

Murali

You're right about COVID-19. Because they're all in their homes, the economy was down, so it was difficult particularly, to be frank, for our womenfolk, who bear a lot of burden. We need to be sensitive to these kinds of matters. That's one big area which I think we need to improve.

I would say beyond that we need to improve on collaboration. The case I spoke to you about involving the person who was shouting at two in the morning, I think I involved at least ten organizations to try and see how we can resolve it, but none of them could solve it on their own because they were all looking at it from their own lenses . . .

MK

So we're talking about openness?

Murali

Collaboration with openness, and then you can perhaps aim for a better impact given the difficulties that they face. I think there needs to be more empathy among our residents as well. And I'm glad to note that when our residents get to know the underlying issues, they tend to be very understanding.

There was one incident during the Circuit Breaker[61] period, where for weeks, there was this complaint of urine dripping down the window of a flat. And again, it's presented as a social disturbance, as if somebody's doing this purposely. *It wasn't done purposely.* It involved an elderly gentleman who was suffering from dementia, and he was using his urinal and, in his state, when it's full, he just empties it. So, you see, that family had to be supported. And how do we do this? We have community involvement because yes, there are neighbours who are angry, but we need to have neighbours who are looking into this and don't deal with it in an accusatory way but a supportive way. If you're doing it in an accusatory way, what will happen then is people will not open their doors, they will not share their problems.

MK

People will get defensive.

Murali

They will get very defensive. *Oh, my dad is okay, no problem.* You know, they—

MK

They go into denial or even omit information.

Murali

Yes, and that makes it a lot more confrontational. But if you have a neighbourhood that is a little bit more accommodating, then I think we can solve these issues better. And we did solve this issue.

MK

Thank you for sharing that with us, Mr Murali. We really loved this conversation.

---

[61] Circuit Breaker refers to the three month nationwide lockdown in Singapore to curb the spread of COVID-19

CHAPTER 8

It Takes a Village to Care for a Person

By Jun Lee, Self-Employed Art Therapist and Art Facilitator

Previously a social worker, Jun Lee shared about the multi-layered challenges that people with mental health conditions face. This reflects on how professionals can be more effective in providing help, and perhaps at the very basic level, how we need to learn how to create a conducive environment by not judging others.

FROM ONE SETTING TO ANOTHER

MK

What got you interested in mental health and suicide prevention?

Jun

Mental health and suicide prevention work was a part of my job scope as a social worker in a family service centre, and later on at a hospital. Inevitably, I met clients and patients with various needs and issues stemming from the stresses they faced in their lives. Oftentimes, they needed a listening ear, and I felt privileged to be entrusted with their personal struggles. While learning on the job, there were also ample opportunities to attend trainings to hone my skills in counselling and empowering my clients and patients to overcome their struggles. Perhaps it was the process of journeying with them and witnessing their transformation and improvement in their wellbeing that kept me going in my work as a social worker. Subsequently, I went on to take up art therapy to value-add to my skills so that I could help them on a deeper level.

Art has always been my passion. Coupled with my experiences as a social worker, I found art therapy to be a marriage of my passion and experience in empowering people. Through art therapy work with my clients, their artwork became the catalyst for them to be more open to expressing and sharing their innermost feelings.

In my pursuit to empower more people to improve their mental health and minimize incidences of suicidal ideation, I decided to move on to be a self-employed art therapist. To date, I have been freelancing as an art therapist cum art facilitator for four years.

HELP AND HELPLESSNESS

MK

Was there an incident that you faced in your career regarding mental health stigmas that shaped your drive and commitment towards the cause in a certain way?

Jun

I recall a case of alcoholism with family violence and financial abuse. I used to think that alcoholics could make the 'right' choices but would rather sacrifice their health, wealth and relationships with their loved ones than quit drinking. In that aspect, I confess to lacking empathy for these people. It wasn't until a particular incident when I encountered an alcoholic patient with a distraught wife and young child. I still remember his countless admissions for his recurrent drinking problem. At each admission, he showed remorse for his addiction and promised to go for rehabilitation at IMH[62]. Each time, his wife would pay his hospitalization fees with her MediSave[63] and was convinced to give him another chance. However, he would revert to his drinking habit each time he was discharged from the hospital. On one occasion, my ex-colleague witnessed him drinking at his void deck with his friends while his young daughter was playing by herself at his side. His wife eventually gave up on him and no longer wanted to pay for his hospitalization fees. The last I heard

[62] IMH: Institute of Mental Health

[63] MediSave is a national medical savings scheme that helps individuals set aside part of their income to pay for their personal or approved dependents' hospitalization, day surgery and certain outpatient expenses, as well as their healthcare needs in old age.

of him was that he had fallen out from his window while drunk and died.

This particular case left me wondering about the success of helping, or if our ways of treatment are effective in helping these patients to quit their addictions. Now, I feel more empathetic towards persons with addictions to alcohol when I relate his addiction with our own individual addictions that we have difficulty quitting—be it food, smoking, or something else.

By stigmatizing an alcoholic as aggressive or financially needy, we as professionals may have unknowingly condemned them as hopeless or people who cannot be helped. The patient I mentioned had me thinking about the way the media often portrays these people and their behaviours, which can influence how their loved ones and society think of them. By focusing on their behaviours that were brought about and aggravated by issues they faced earlier in their lives, we failed to understand them and their needs. Thinking of this particular case got me to be more reflective in my subsequent work with people. Whenever I am stuck on a case in assisting a person in embracing change for the better, I make a more conscious effort to put myself in the shoes of that person to understand him or her better first.

WHAT DO YOU REALLY NEED?

MK

Based on your personal experiences over the years, what do you think are the most common things that people struggle with when it comes to mental health?

Jun

They struggle with coming to an acceptance of their condition, their situation, and the issues they face. They also struggle with how society in general views them. Everyone wants to have a sense of belonging without being judged by others. People suffering from mental illnesses very often find themselves fighting a lonely battle. They find themselves in various difficult situations—from finding it difficult to share with their loved ones what they're going through, to feeling that the people around them do not empathize with their struggles. They could also be in denial about their own conditions. Many of them believe that there is no way out of their predicament, which often leads to suicidal tendencies. A good example is work-induced stress, which often leads to depression. People hesitate to confide in their colleagues or immediate superiors for fear of being labelled as incompetent. Our societal views on mental illnesses create a poor environment for people to break out of their mental struggles. Everyone must be kinder and understand that mental illness can befall anyone, and it is not an illness that befalls only people who are mentally 'weak'. From the caregiver aspect, witnessing loved ones showing early signs of mental upset and brushing it off tends to lead to the worsening of their conditions.

MK

Quite a real-time issue that's happening in our society right now. Oftentimes when people finally start looking for help, it's usually too late by then. And I think some people have difficulty connecting with or understanding people struggling with mental health. What advice would you have for them?

Jun

I think we can start by learning how to detect certain signs. People who might be struggling with their own mental health issues often have a change in behaviour. They might begin to say or do things that are different from their usual selves. If they become very temperamental or aggressive and start exhibiting behaviours that are different from their usual selves, it could be early signs of mental illness.

A great starting point would be for loved ones to initiate conversations with questions. *How are you? I noticed that you seem bothered by something. Is there anything you wish to share? What can I do to brighten your day?* Simple questions like these could encourage people to share and feel more comfortable coming forward to talk or get help.

THERE'S ALWAYS A CHOICE

Jun

I have had friends telling me how envious they are of me being a freelancer. They share about their stresses at work and being unable to leave due to financial constraints and limited choices. In reality, many people do not have the luxury of living their lives the way they want it, let alone set up a career doing what they are really passionate about. Most people in Singapore are burdened by financial obligations which trap them in a job that, while providing them a comfortable lifestyle, doesn't really fulfil them.

MK

And that's quite a pity because the human spirit isn't getting fuelled. The fire inside the belly gets smaller every day because they're in a place that's not aligned with them.

We spend one-third of our day-to-day life on our jobs. That's eight hours a day. Those are the main productive waking hours we have, and we spend them on a job we don't love. In the next one-third of our day, most of us don't have the energy to do the things that matter to us. We're drained from a full day of work. And the last one-third we spend sleeping. So technically, the only time when we're working consciously is during that first one-third, which is why people tend to associate their identities with their job titles. That's why, when you go to networking events, people always say, *Hello, I'm a banker. I'm a social worker.* People will always introduce themselves as their job titles, but the problem is, we are not our titles.

Jun

I think it's also how we're being brought up. Our own expectations that arise due to societal norms also influence the way we think, how we behave, and that shapes our perception towards mental health.

MK

The funny thing is sometimes we chase after all these expectations without recognizing what is important to us. Your parents once told you it's important to be rich, therefore you spend your life chasing after that, for example. Or because you thought that being rich means happiness. I can list down a lot of the different examples I've seen throughout the years. It really does not matter what titles we carry. Ultimately, it is really who we are inside.

Jun

Indeed! We can have all the frameworks and systems in place to help people suffering from mental illnesses. However, without a caring and accepting society, people suffering from mental health conditions will still feel stigmatized and find it hard to break free from their chains.

Everyone born in Singapore is blessed with good education, governance and social security. Let us give back to society by being more caring, generous, and loving as individuals.

CHAPTER 9

Tapping into the Coffeeshop Conversations

By Eric Chua, Parliamentary Secretary, Ministry of Social and Family Development & Ministry of Culture, Community and Youth

Drawing from his experiences working with people and communities, Eric Chua shares that mental health stigmas are a result of a lack of understanding, which shapes our beliefs and attitudes. In order to tackle stigma effectively, we need to create conversations that enlighten people on what mental health really is, and allow an exchange of ideas so that beliefs and attitudes start changing.

TAPPING INTO THE COFFEESHOP CONVERSATIONS

MK

As a leader, what are some of the mental health challenges that you've observed when you're on the ground?

Eric

I just had a series of meetings the past two nights, actually. Meetings with my community leaders, and grassroots leaders. One of the key things that I've been asking them to look into, especially in the upcoming month ahead, is the mental wellbeing of our residents in Queenstown, especially for seniors who are living alone. Because the average age in Queenstown is older than the national average, we do have quite a sizable number of seniors in the town. Some of them live alone because their children got married and left Queenstown. Some of them, because of family circumstances, they're living alone. They're at that stage of their lives where sometimes what they look forward to on a daily basis is going to the *kopitiam*[64], the hawker centre, not only for their cup of coffee, but also more importantly, to meet up with their 'now loved ones' who are their neighbourhood friends and fellow uncles and aunties living in the precinct. Some of them will even travel from different precincts and gather at, say, for instance, Tanglin Halt. And then in Tanglin Halt, we have another dimension of things because Tanglin Halt as you know, it's now undergoing probably the largest SERS[65] migration in Singapore's history. We're slowly moving residents out from Tanglin Halt, which is an old estate with its own charms, into the redeveloped Margaret Drive. Because of the COVID situation and how construction

---

[64] Kopitiam: Singapore hawker centre

[65] SERS: Selective En-Bloc Redevelopment Scheme

has been delayed and whatnot, there's uncertainty, especially for residents living in Tanglin Halt. There are delays, for sure, in the process of getting the keys to their new HDB[66] flats. So quite a bit of uncertainty for this group of residents in Tanglin Halt, many of whom are elderly residents.

Before the restrictions[67] came in, when I was having morning coffee with the residents, oftentimes I hear questions: *Oh, when will the new Margaret Drive blocks be ready? How long will the delays be?* A lot is going on, and there's a lot on the minds of many people. It's good to be connected to the conversations in the coffee shops, in the hawker centres so that you're actually plugged in to the collective psyche of the folks, and you sort of understand where they come from, where their anxieties stem from, and I think many of these would have a bearing on their state of mental wellbeing because we're talking about uncertainty and movement. And also, there's a bit of that life stage effect that we're talking about. Seniors are living alone, and we have to consider how we can tap on the role of the community to provide some form of kinship, some form of friendship, and some form of relationship that fuels these old folks on a day-to-day basis.

HOW COME WE DIDN'T PICK THIS UP EARLIER?

MK

As you're working with people on the ground, what are some of the mental health stigmas you see happening?

Eric

If you talk about mental health stigma specifically, those are best illustrated by some numbers. I talked about these numbers on

[66] HDB: Housing Development Board

[67] This interview was conducted during the Phase 2 (Heightened Alert) period.

various platforms before, in Parliament as well. There was a survey that was done, I think it was the Singapore Mental Health Study,[68] that was initiated in 2016. What was interesting about that survey is that one in seven Singaporeans above eighteen had experienced a mental health condition in their lifetime. Although one in seven is not a huge number, it shows that it's quite prevalent. But despite that, we still see attitudes to mental health conditions being not as ideal as they should be.

And here's where some other statistics, which I always go back to, are in order. There was a Study on Public Attitudes towards Persons with Mental Health Conditions in Singapore[69] done by NCSS[70] in 2017. It revealed that more than five in ten are not willing to live nearby or work with a person with a mental health condition. To me, that is testimony of fear—fear that probably stems from the lack of understanding, possibly, that people still might have, surrounding mental health conditions and people with mental health conditions. Now, there are a couple of other statistics, which I think are also very telling, from NCSS' Public Attitudes Study in 2017. One in three expressed the view that one of the main causes of mental health conditions is a lack of self-discipline and willpower. That's quite a sizable number, and it reflects a misunderstanding of mental health conditions and how it comes about. Just one last statistic from this same study, which is again, very telling. One in five feels that if you're somebody with mental health conditions, then you shouldn't be given any

---

[68] M. Subramaniam, E. Abdin, J. A. Vaingankar, S. Shafie, B.Y. Chua, R. Sambasivam, Y. J. Zhang, et al., 'Tracking the Mental Health of a Nation: Prevalence and Correlates of Mental Disorders in the Second Singapore Mental Health Study', *Epidemiology and Psychiatric Sciences* 29, 2020: e29. doi:10.1017/S2045796019000179.

[69] 'NCSS Launches First Nation-Wide Campaign to Fight Mental Health Stigma', National Council of Social Service, 2018, National Council of Social Service, https://www.ncss.gov.sg/docs/default-source/ncss-press-release-doc/mh-anti-stigma-campaign-launch-release-pdf.pdf.

[70] NCSS: National Council of Social Service

responsibility. That to me, that's, *wow*. That's a huge statement to make! Because what do we then do with people with mental health conditions? And to me, that also speaks volumes of how mental health conditions are misunderstood. Because people with mental health conditions, be it depressive disorders or other disorders, actually day-to-day for a large part of their lives, they can be quite high-functioning for a large part of their day-to-day lives. And that's also why some of these conditions are quite hard to detect.

During the budget debate in Parliament, I talked about a young lady that I spoke to. Her name is Courtney. Courtney is now a twenty-year-old young woman, very confident. If you see her, you'll feel that *wow, this is a confident lady that has done well.* She got admitted to a local institution, quite a good one. She did well academically and got a scholarship for her studies. But she was a person with mental health conditions. And her problem then, as she looked back, was that she didn't recognize that she had those conditions, and not even the people around her recognized that she's got those conditions. Because she's just telling herself, *I don't think I'm somebody who can suffer from this. I don't think I am actually suffering. I'm doing well. How could I be somebody who's suffering from mental health conditions?* And she said things like *everyone hates me, but I don't deserve sympathy*. And there were thoughts that were running through her mind. And you know what? For her case, she was so affected by it that she gave up school in Singapore. She went to New Zealand, enrolled in a vocational school, and she had a major breakdown in New Zealand. That's when she had to seek help. And incidentally, as she was seeking help, she was diagnosed with depressive disorders alongside other conditions, and it was only then that she realized: *How come I didn't pick this up earlier?* Or, *how come people around me also didn't pick this up earlier?* Because the people around her, her teachers, her peers, couldn't quite understand why her attendance was dropping, or why she was having issues when she was once a role model. I think the lack of understanding, part of which feeds the stigma, is still a major hurdle that we are dealing with in Singapore.

GUIDING OUR BEHAVIOURS AND SPEECH WITH OUR CORE VALUES

MK

What do you think is causing all these phenomena?

Eric

[heavily sighing]

I think all of us, throughout life, are actually shaped by our experiences, and as we go about life, we are sometimes told what to think, how to think. And how we behave, meaning what we say and what we do: those outwardly expressions are more often than not a manifestation of our attitudes. At a deeper level, our beliefs, and at an even deeper level, our values. So, values-wise, I'd like to think that humans, Singaporeans especially, share the values of wanting to care for each other. I truly believe that.

But in terms of the beliefs which actually shape our attitudes, which shape our behaviour and speech; that's where I think we can change it up a little bit. Because the lack of understanding surrounding mental health conditions causes us to behave in a certain way. And oftentimes, those sets of misconceptions are also present in the people with mental health conditions themselves. How many times did you actually feel, *Eh I'm feeling so stressed, I'm feeling so down, and I need help*, but your own next statement is *eh, but I don't want to tell anyone in my life. I don't want to tell my family members. I don't want to tell my boyfriend, girlfriend. I don't want to tell my husband, wife.* Why? Because you fear that you'll be a burden to them. Because you think, *Hey, they already have a lot in their lives, do I want to add one more load in the wheelbarrow they're carrying?* I think that's probably also a very culturally Asian way of thinking. I feel that way. So that's what

I think: a lack of understanding and the way we interact with the members in the community probably accounts for a large part of why we hesitate to seek help in these contexts.

MK

And you're saying that all these little things kind of stack up and form stigmas down the road?

Eric

All these little things kind of stack up, and they influence how we behave, and influence how we react to each other. And we need to dig a little bit deeper into our attitudes, into our beliefs, to start changing things that we used to think should be the way, that we used to think is right. Only then will we start seeing changes in our behaviours and in our speech. And that really speaks to how we probably have not quite understood the problem of mental health conditions as we should have.

MK

Got it. Part of it is really about going back to ourselves, looking into what really matters to us, into who we are as a person. Our value systems, what matters, and our belief systems as well. Part of it is about self-enquiry, about questioning what's real for us. What's our truth? More than anything else.

So how do you think we can begin to encourage self-awareness in people? Because, for the most part, we tend to look outwards for answers. Every time there are problems, the easiest thing to do is to look outwards. But what does it take for individuals to look into themselves?

Eric

I think you've just mentioned the answer yourself! Because remember I mentioned, first of all, the outer rings of the onion are speech and behaviours, a little bit deeper are attitudes, a little bit deeper are beliefs, but at the core of it all are our values.

I believe many of us have good values. Values of love for fellow mankind, values of love for this earth that we treasure, value of being generous with the people around us. We just have to connect with those good old values and let them shine through. Because while I don't believe that we are in a state where we don't treat each other well because of malice, I think that currently, we're not necessarily thinking about the way we should think about mental health and other folks with mental health conditions, not because of our value system, but because of the lack of understanding. Understanding that shapes our beliefs and attitudes.

MK

Got it. Got it.

Eric

Understanding mental health conditions, that's what we've been trying to do—not just within the government—but we have a lot of ground-up groups that have been trying to do this. I think in your exhibition, in the last round, that's what you're trying to do as well, to get people to be in touch with their inner selves and to have a conversation surrounding mental health and its place in our society. How we, as a society, can deal with mental health conditions, and how we, as a collective, can help people with mental health conditions. Those conversations need to be had and it all begins with conversations, because conversations would then feed into how we perceive things and how we believe things to be. And that's why we have so many things like NCSS doing the Beyond the Label movement. Once you start a topic, you have an exchange of ideas, and that's when beliefs and attitudes start changing.

And we need to have conversations not just in the community at large, but specifically in schools and in workplaces. We need to have a better understanding by employers, by students, peers in schools as well. A lot more needs to be done. And that's also part of the big reason we had set up the Youth Mental Wellbeing Network. That was started last year, and we now have about 1,500 members from different walks of life and different life experiences who are passionate about mental wellbeing. They're brainstorming, co-creating projects that they feel they could work together on, and our folks in MSF[71], MOE[72] and MOH[73] are matching them to resources and all that.

And talking about resources, I believe we are in a better state than before. What we need to do is to bring about awareness to people who might need these resources so that they know where to seek professional help. It's also a matter of clearing some misconceptions. For instance, *If I seek professional help, I'll be forever blackmarked.* That's not the case. Most of the services provided are anonymous. We need to clear out some of these older ways or more traditional ways of thinking in favour of seeking help.

YOU'RE NOT THE ONLY MAN ON THE ISLAND

MK

What would be your message to individuals out there, to the general public, about mental health?

Eric

To those who are possibly feeling or know that they need help in areas of mental health, it's key to note that it's really, *really* okay not to be okay. It's cliché, but it's worth repeating.

---

[71] MSF: Ministry of Social and Family Development

[72] MOE: Ministry of Education

[73] MOH: Ministry of Health

Apart from knowing that it's okay not to be okay, it is also important to know that you are hardly alone. Remember, one in seven. So, in a room of thirty, that's about at least three or four other people with mental health conditions in the same room. And it's really more prevalent than one thinks it is, because the sense of being alone, that *hey, mental health conditions, probably I'm the only bloke on this island that's feeling stranded, that is feeling lost*, isn't true.

You're not alone. Reach out, seek help, and most of all, you're not weak if you seek help. You're strong because you recognize that you have an issue you need to address, and you're addressing it head-on.

I have another message for those of us who might come across friends or family members who might need help in this area. If we do come across a social media post or somebody in their daily speech where you feel that something's not quite right: my message to this group of people is that you don't have to be a superhero to be somebody who renders help. Sometimes just lending a listening ear or simply being present, lending a shoulder, will help a lot already. And we do want folks to be more sensitive and react faster to such nuances or sentiments that you might pick up. In the realm of psychological first aid, we always advocate the three Ls—Look, Listen, and Link. *Look* out for behaviours and speech. *Listen* to what the person is saying. *Link* that person to potential resources that he or she might need. If the person requires more assistance or professional help, perhaps a psychologist or psychiatrist. So, look, listen, link. That's a useful mantra to remember!

CHAPTER 10

Invest and Commit to Helping Someone Else

By Cheryl Chan, Member of Parliament (East Coast GRC), Advisor to Fengshan GROs

Mental health in the community may come about in the form of neighbourly disputes, noise pollution, or even a hoarding issue, and it takes a very tolerant neighbourhood to be able to empathize with the mental health stresses present within families. Cheryl Chan talks about how it takes a high level of commitment and time to continuously build relationships and trust with others in order to help them in the long run.

RAISING AWARENESS AND TOLERANCE IN THE COMMUNITY

MK

Now, you've been on the ground working with people for a very long time. As you go around meeting residents, what are some of the mental health stigmas that you've observed?

Cheryl

Many of these stigmas show up in neighbourly disputes. For example, it might be very simple things like noise complaints, with people asking, *Why do people always drag things on the floor?* What people don't recognize is that sometimes in certain families, the individual is actually struggling with a mental health condition. Some are seniors who live on their own, and it's hard for the domestic helper to manage their condition.

Another example is families who have kids with special needs. It takes very tolerant neighbours as well as a community to be able to support these individuals. They're not sure why kids constantly throw tantrums in certain ways, and it actually does cause mental stress to others living with and around them.

I've met families with members who have hoarding problems. The children, or even the spouse, live through it for a long period of time under suppressed conditions, and they just don't know how to deal with it. Whatever that's within the flat space is supposed to be a common area for them, and they should be able to freely move about. But sometimes they do not get that freedom, and children have reached out because they felt stressed living and growing up in those environments, and eventually, it does have an impact on their own mental health as well. They have to go through psychiatric assessments because they either grew up literally in the environment, or they felt coerced into a particular position that is not their choice.

We have to raise awareness of such issues. We can't expect everyone to accept this, but at least they have to see how they can reach out and have a higher tolerance or understand that there would be mental stresses within families. Parents go through it. Some working parents have seniors at home to take care of, have kids they have to manage, and it does cause marital problems as well.

BUILDING RELATIONSHIPS AND TRUST IN THE COMMUNITY

MK

What are some interventions that we can implement, including whatever that we are currently already doing, that can effectively resolve these situations?

Cheryl

I do not think there will be one single solution that will resolve all these. Whenever it comes to individual or family circumstances, it's complex, because family conditions change. Individual needs, their life stages, and what they go through also vary. At least what can be done along the way, or what we can continue improving first, is to be aware of all these different combinations or different circumstances and situations that arise. The reason there's stigmatization is that people always have their own biases, and they put their own assumptions and values against others. I think it needs individual self-reflection as well. If you were put in that situation, how would you counter it? If you were the individual experiencing it, what would you do?

Another way is to form support networks for these individuals. Sometimes when situations get complex or complicated, the community will try to distance themselves from the individuals or the families. They will say, *This is a problematic family*. They know there's a hoarding problem, but they choose to ignore them as long as it doesn't affect their life. They will only complain if it affects them. Of course, that being said, all these things are mutual. It doesn't mean the individual will want to step forward for help. Some people with mental stress do not want to disclose or even acknowledge the fact that they are in that situation or have conditions. I wouldn't say all are under self-denial, but some simply refuse all help, whether it's because of pride or whatever reason. We can't force things upon them, so we have to just try to offer that platform or even the aid and hopefully, they will be willing to step forward at some point. But I think all this starts with building relationships and trust.

From a policy angle, any policy that you implement tends to transcend many different disciplines, and therefore, we need to look at the most immediate need this individual or family has, which is why we have all these social service workers stepping out to help. Sometimes multi-ministries or multi-agencies actually come out to support just one particular family. Because after addressing the issue with, say, the children, the parents will then experience different problems, and so on and so forth, and it creates a vicious cycle. Like I said, it can't be just a single solution. It won't work because some of these are not just about finances; it's beyond that.

MK

When you say beyond that, what are these factors?

Cheryl

I've seen this individual who got bullied in school because she's been under all these suppressed emotional conditions. She did not easily relate or talk about her issues to people, and her neighbour became her close friend, but there's only so much the neighbour can do. So, the next natural thing for her was to reach out to her siblings, but not all siblings share that same warm, cohesive relationship. Sometimes you may not even get support within the family itself, and therefore the need for an external party like social workers to step in to see how they can help, because the immediate concern around youths is not just about their education or studies. It's also about how they can grow up well and have the right moral guidance and values, because some of them do not have strong communication with their parents and did not receive that proper upbringing. That's what I meant by, it's beyond just financial aid to the individual or families.

PAY IT FORWARD TO HELP SOMEONE

MK

There are a lot of common themes around 'connection' that keep coming up as you're describing all these things that you observe. How can people deepen their connections, their relationships with people around them, and even with themselves?

Cheryl

That's never an easy task to achieve! Because I think connections, building trust, and deepening relationships take time and commitment. It's also the investment on every front. Whether it's emotional investment or time investment, something has to give way, right? You have to make sacrifices in order to commit to certain things, and if this individual, for example, is not even your family member, would you make the effort to do it? I think this is what people always question. People these days are very busy. They have many things to juggle in life on their own before they even think of someone else. I think being able to pay it forward is another aspect that we hope we can inculcate in our younger generation.

MK

Got it. Now, if there could be a message you would like to share to the public about mental health, about connections, what would that be?

Cheryl

One is for people who are going through mental stress, or are beginning to see symptoms of their own mental health conditions, to speak up and seek help. They should not shy away from it or bottle it up, because all this gets accumulated over time, and it has long-term implications if they've always been suffering from a particular condition for too long.

The other one would be for people to invest and commit to helping someone else, in whatever way it may be. Sometimes you may not pick it up immediately as a mental-health-related issue. But it all starts from a trigger point. If you feel that an individual you know, even your siblings, family members, or even neighbours are going through a certain phase or difficult situation in their life, take the effort to understand and put yourself in their shoes and see how you can provide moral and mental support, because not everyone needs another individual to solve the issues for them. They just need that companionship and support in life.

CHAPTER 11

Mental Health in the Migrant Workers' Space

By Jolene, Volunteer in the Migrant Workers' Space

COVID-19 cast a spotlight on the living conditions of migrant workers, and it sparked a conversation about the effects of physical space on one's mental wellbeing. The pandemic also created a lot of uncertainty among migrant workers, who had to deal with changing work and living restrictions. Jolene reflects on a year of volunteering in the migrant workers' space, and how Singaporeans can create a more welcoming environment for our migrant brothers.

GOING THROUGH THE PANDEMIC IN A FOREIGN LAND

Si Qi

Can you tell us more about who you are and what you do?

Jolene

My main interest is mental health. I'm a current volunteer involved in the migrant space. My personal interest is also in mental health so I focus on the mental health of migrant workers too.

I got involved in the migrant worker space last year. Through the past year, we've kind of pushed through a lot of different things. I think at one point you could see the mental health come up because we decided to do some projects surrounding mental health, which is really important with the ongoing restrictions.

Si Qi

How was it like to work with the migrant workers during the Circuit Breaker[74] period? I mean, we all heard how many cases were coming out from the dorms, and their living conditions were exposed. I think everybody was concerned about how crammed the spaces were, and how it doesn't really seem like a very conducive space to live in for a very long period of time, with or without COVID. What was it like looking into that?

Jolene

I don't think I was very involved in the migrant worker space before either, so I can't say I really knew much. I also came to know more about it during the COVID-19 period. Working with

[74] Circuit Breaker refers to the three month nationwide lockdown in Singapore to curb the spread of COVID-19

migrant worker organizations gave me an opportunity to meet migrant brothers and really understand more about what they were going through and seeing how, even when they were moved out into less cramped spaces, there is still that base level of lack of privacy in cramped spaces that takes a toll on their mental health. And that's something very easy to not think about when you're not in that position, when you're not exposed to this. But once you are, I think it becomes necessary to put into perspective and want to do something about.

Just imagine you or me, having to share a room with one sibling. You're already so irritated, and you want your own personal space. Then imagine a room of that size shared with five or ten people. I think that's quite an accessible way to think about it. People can understand how that is stressful, especially when they were also being restricted during Circuit Breaker. In some sense, there was an understanding of the living conditions, and that's also why people responded the way they did in supporting and believing that there was a need for change.

But, slightly off tangent, I do feel that as time has passed, at this point, there has been a slight pivot and lessening of support because we're at the point where migrant worker stories have saturated the news to some extent. People are tired of hearing about it, or just don't care any more. People are like, *Oh, new dorms have been built, some have been moved out, they got to stay in hotels for a while*. Or saying *now that they've started working again, there's nothing wrong any more, they should have nothing bothering them any more*. But if you really think about it, there's so much that plays a part, and there are still so many living and movement issues that they still have now. If you decrease from ten people to six people a room, it's still too many people per room for any kind of conducive living environment. Especially those who live in huge PBDs, where there's just so many people.

Si Qi

What's a PBD?

Jolene

Purpose-built dormitory. So those are the biggest, with a few thousand people living in those dorms. There are some rooms with ten people per room in double-decker beds. The placement of it is like, there are two beds on the side, and then a one-metre space, and the middle two are connected, so it's four people. Imagine sleeping side by side in the next bunk bed with no screen in between at all. There's absolutely zero privacy; there's no personal space. Your friend can sleep and move his hand across and it's in your face like that. Those kinds of things are still an issue, I think.

Si Qi

Could you share a little more about the mental health conditions of migrant workers during the height of Circuit Breaker? Because there were news articles in the media about suicide cases and suicide attempts.

Jolene

During the COVID-19 period, we understood from a lot of our migrant friends that there were widespread mental health issues. And that's so understandable: it must have been extremely stressful to feel so uncertain and anxious about your job security. Some migrant brothers also had no idea where they were going or how long they'd be staying in a place. Also, some workers were moved to hotels, whether it was for quarantine or just to be decanted. And they sometimes stayed there for a few months, which led to a lot of feelings of isolation. Even if the workers were healthy, the hotel didn't have any common areas and maybe not even windows!. Can you imagine not having fresh air for months?

What added to the anxiety among the workers was that they weren't receiving any information about the COVID situation in Singapore because of the language barriers. And I think that's why, during that time, there were some Facebook pages that came up that were run by migrant workers to translate and provide information, even from the MOM[75] and MOH[76] circulars, because they didn't really understand what was going on, and all the information they got was in English, and not all of them can speak English. And with that complete lack of information, they didn't know where to go. For the hotlines, a lot of them called just because they didn't know how else to get in contact with anybody. They didn't need anything specific; they just needed information. They wanted somebody to talk to and to find out what was going on. And that really shows the lack of resources available to them, and that really took a toll on them.

I think you can have all the resources in the world. There were so many good hotlines that people were trying to set up in their languages, but if the workers don't know about them, then it defeats the purpose. And I think that can be seen as quite reflective of Singapore and Singapore's mental health scene in general. I think a lot of people don't know about the really good mental health services available. Like even I just recently found out some counselling services like SAMH[77] can be completely free!

Si Qi

Wow, I actually didn't know that either!

---

[75] MOM: Ministry of Manpower

[76] MOH: Ministry of Health

[77] SAMH: Singapore Association of Mental Health

MENTAL HEALTH ISN'T JUST ABOUT THE SYMPTOMS AND DISORDERS

Si Qi

Let's talk more about mental health stigmas. To put it into the context of migrant workers in Singapore, what do you think are some mental health stigmas that are prevalent in the community about receiving help or getting help?

Jolene

Actually, a lot of the migrant workers that I've spoken to don't necessarily directly talk about it, the same way that a lot of Singaporeans don't directly talk about it. But a lot of the leaders in the migrant worker community have been very eager to champion migrant worker health issues. They want other people to know about it, they want other people to understand, and they especially want Singaporeans to understand. For example, they want us to know how their employer treats them, the instability around their money and their jobs, that all these things play a part in their general mental wellbeing. I think that's the focus for a lot of them. There are migrant workers with genuine mental health conditions, but I think what we've seen so far is that a lot of the time, it is situational and basic mental-wellness-related.

I do think that it's a big part of mental health, and that's the thing that people don't understand. Mental health isn't just *oh this person has depression, this person is schizophrenic.* I'm not saying that there aren't situations where mental illness is due to physiological reasons. But speaking about mental health in general—not just mental disorders, it starts from, *I have these things that impact my mental wellbeing* and *if my mental wellbeing is impacted too much, then it becomes a more serious situation.* Because it's just like physical health! When it deteriorates too much, it does have an impact. It's something that people need to understand, that you don't have to have a mental illness to need to support your mental health or want to support or manage your mental health better. And I think that's something that migrant workers do talk about, or have been wanting to talk about.

But at this point, and rightly so, there are a lot of other non-mental health issues that they want to cover and so when they talk about it and share their experiences, many a time it's about feeling helpless because of a certain situation. A lot of systemic change needs to happen to alleviate a lot of these things. It's like how in Singapore, our children are super stressed because of the way our education system is built, but there's only so much that you can do by teaching them better tips for meditation, or wellbeing, or how to take a break. The rest of it has to be actually changing the system to allow everyone to benefit from having less pressure.

JUST SAY HI

Si Qi

I think that's really true. What do you think we can do now to support the migrant workers, both from an individual and a community standpoint?

Jolene

I guess one of the most basic things that our migrant workers always say, and it's something so simple, is just to say *hi*. Just acknowledge them, acknowledge their presence, acknowledge them as people. I've often heard that many migrant brothers feel like their humanity is not remembered. And this is a very basic step that shows that they are welcome, and they are allowed to be in our spaces as an equal. I think that does and can play a big part in improving even the most basic aspect of mental wellbeing, because you don't want to be somewhere where you're not welcome. And I think especially now, because of COVID, there's a lot of fear as well because at one point there were so many cases in the dorms. It became almost like a justification for being scared of them or wanting to stay away from them. And that created an even bigger barrier and made the othering of migrant workers so much more prominent. They're not a small community, but our actions could make them feel so small and unwanted. The most basic step we can take is to just acknowledge them.

The next step would be to approach them and treat them as equals. I'm happy that with my experiences with different migrant worker organizations, it's always a partnership because we don't always want to have the dynamic where *oh, migrants are such underprivileged people; oh, we need to help*. We don't want every single time we interact with them to be like, *what can I give you, what can I do for you, can I donate something to you?* Because that's not always how they want to be treated. For example, if you were speaking to someone you genuinely treated as a friend, you wouldn't start every single conversation asking what you can do or give to them, right? Just because you have less than somebody else doesn't mean that you don't have enough, or don't have pride or dignity, or that you don't have the ability to support yourself. A lot of migrant workers have said this too. They said, 'We appreciate the money, we appreciate the food, we appreciate the gifts, but what we would appreciate is if you would champion for us to get more courses so we can go further in our career, so we can earn more money, so that you don't have to give us the food, we can afford the food ourselves.' And that's a basic thing to feel. If you have to rely on the help of somebody else, I don't think that that's very good for your own self-image sometimes too. And I think that's a systemic thing that will be hard to change, but that's something that we've heard many times as well. I think it's such a good point. A lot of the migrant workers with mid-tier positions get to go for supervisor courses and things like that so that they get to be supervisors of their migrant brothers. But the job progression obviously, without the education, is different. Some of them go for engineering diplomas, but not all of them have those opportunities. And with those opportunities, there could be so much more that they could do, and that's what they want more than anything, I think.

Si Qi

It also speaks about this very nonchalant Singaporean attitude where I mean, it's not just migrant workers, but we may not even talk to our neighbours. As a society, we're so fast paced, we're already so busy as it is, there is no time to slow down and talk to somebody on the street.

Jolene

I think the same. There are so many people around us, but it's so easy to feel disconnected because you're not really connecting to other people. You know when you're in other countries and the people are very friendly, you'll just stop on the street and have a chat with people you barely know. That's not the kind of thing I would ever expect to happen in Singapore.

And that also translates into how our migrant brothers feel. Previously, they were sharing with me that back home in Bangladesh, they have a very strong *kampong* spirit[78], a neighbourly and friendly culture. Everybody that they see, when they travel around, it's like getting a Grab and talking to your driver. They'll be like *oh, eh brother!* and they'll talk to them the entire time. They'll actually sit down and have a chat with them. And some Singaporeans will do that in a Grab, fine, but a lot of us won't, right? We just—

---

[78] *Kampong* spirit refers to a neighbourly and friendly culture

Si Qi

Use our phones.

Jolene

The entire time. And so, coming from a culture like that, it's even more jarring for them to be so ignored. To them, it's like the next level of disconnection here.

Si Qi

Yeah! The level of disconnect in Singapore at least is quite high lah, which is why we are called *ThisConnect* . . .

Si Qi

Because we're disconnected not only from each other but also from ourselves. We don't even know what we are feeling and what we are experiencing. And most of the time, we opt to sweep things under the carpet and just deal with it that way, but they don't really go away, do they?

CULTURAL NUANCES: WHEN FREE MEALS GOT MISMATCHED

Si Qi

Anyway, you were mentioning a little bit about their life back in Bangladesh, and I think there are a lot of misconceptions or a lack of understanding that Singaporeans have about migrant workers, like maybe they are less educated. What are some of the biggest misconceptions that people might have?

Jolene

Some migrant workers actually have university degrees. It's just that when they come to Singapore, they have to do a different job. There are so many other things.

I think culturally, we won't even understand the difference in their culture unless we really get to know them. And it's quite funny. I was hearing from them about the differences in culture. When the migrant workers were provided free meals, be it from donors or their hospital meals, sometimes they were only provided Tamil food, and everyone from Bangladesh didn't want to eat the Tamil food. And those from Tamil Nadu didn't want to eat the Bangladeshi food. So, there's the whole issue about that because they have specific tastes as well right? Or remembering the need for Halal or vegetarian meals. Like, we mean well, but there are more levels we can take to understand them, and food is such a big comfort for us as Singaporeans and I think it'll be so important for us to understand that it is in other cultures too. And if we can appreciate that, I think it is very helpful to everybody.

There was one point during the lockdown when one of my migrant brothers posted a different food photo of something that he missed from back home. Because he had COVID, he was in the hospital eating really bad food, like really *bad* food. And every day he would post the food that he misses, and he'll have hundreds of comments from other migrant brothers like, *oh ya, that was so good, the one here was the best,* or *I remember I had this from my family.* Those things create very positive reminders for them about the things that they miss. And if we could share in that with them, I think it'll help us to build our understanding with them in a way that would bolster everyone's mental health.

Si Qi

I think maybe some people will feel that it's difficult to connect with someone from such a different culture, or they don't even know how to. In your experience, what is it really like to connect with someone else from these very different backgrounds?

Jolene

I think it's the simple things. I guess the basis of it is to get past that mental block of treating them as somebody you need to help, because you wouldn't approach a friend like that. When you hang out with your friends, you just talk about things you have in common, things that you both enjoy. That's how all friendships are built. Like, you're not friends with everybody. It's kind of the same thing, right? You're not going to be friends with every single migrant worker you meet because we have different personalities.

But it has to come from a different level than approaching a beneficiary or helping somebody in need. And I think that's a dynamic I want to keep, because it's the respect and the understanding that we are equals. I don't always need to help you. If you want my help, you tell me, or I'll ask you if you would mind, the way you ask a friend, for instance, *You said you're struggling with this, would you mind if I helped you?* That's the way you approach a friend. It's not an immediate *I can do it, I can solve the issue for you, I'm helping you.*

KNOWING WHO TO HELP AND WHEN TO HELP

Si Qi

So it's a level of consensus that we need to reach even with giving help.

Jolene

It depends on where you're coming from, right? There are a lot of initiatives that allow Singaporeans to do things to help migrant workers, but Singaporeans might want to help without necessarily wanting to be their friends. And that's fair, there's nothing wrong with that. For example, so many people donated to *It's Raining Raincoats,* and they got to do that amazing thing where they brought our migrant workers to the Singapore Flyer. That's something that the migrant workers treasure just as much, but it's completely different from you saying that you want to be friends with a migrant worker and all you do is ask how you can help them.

And I guess there are two very different things. For example, our migrant brothers have been very vocal about how they want to attend courses and how they want help with specific things. And they keep telling us, *Please tell your Singaporeans just say hi to us, it will make us happy*. It's like if I told you, *I really appreciate when you text me before you call me because I don't like just being called,* it's the kind of courtesy that you do for a friend when they request it of you. It's not just you helping or doing what you think is best for them. I guess that's the essence of what I'm trying to say. It's very different when you're trying to be their friend versus trying to help them, because trying to help them doesn't necessarily mean you're helping them in the way they want to be helped.

For example, all these different people donating care packets to the migrant workers. What if they get items they don't want to or can't eat? What are they going to do with them? It's also important to understand their needs.

Si Qi

I think that's something to think about, even for our everyday relationships. Sometimes when somebody is feeling down or feeling stressed and you want to help, but that person is not receptive, sometimes people will feel very offended: *Why don't you want me to help you? Why don't you want to get help? Why don't you want to get better?* But we forget to think about what the other person needs.

Jolene

Yeah! I do have quite a few friends who struggle with mental health, but I won't step in unless I think they're in a dire condition and I need to act right now. Otherwise, I stop, I wait, and I text them to see what I can do for them, how I can support them, and I wait for them to tell me what they want. Sometimes they'll say, *No, but maybe I want to call you later,* and then I'll just keep my phone on standby in case they want to hang out, or if they say, *Actually can you come pick me up right now*, then I'll be there and I'll do that.

But especially when you're going through something, it's very hard for people who've never experienced that to understand that sometimes it's too overwhelming to have someone offer help, and sometimes it isn't what's helpful at that moment. For example, you're having a panic attack. Not only do you have to balance the panic attack you're having, but you have to think about some friend who you don't want to offend by being rude to them. And that's something that Singaporeans don't really understand, and I feel that psychoeducation can help with that. There are a lot of Instagram accounts right now that do try to educate on different symptoms, different conditions, and how you can support. And that's very good because that equips younger Singaporeans at least with the basics to be able to take the steps to phrase things in a way that can be more beneficial to those who are experiencing distress.

But at the same time, it's not enough, lah. There's always more that needs to be done. There's also a need to understand when you need to give someone space. It's the same with everything, with migrant workers or anyone else, that how much you can help somebody is really dependent on how much they want to be helped. In the context of migrant workers, there are two extremes. Some workers are like, *I don't want any help, just let me do my job, I just want to support my family*. But you have the other spectrum of people who are vocal in asking for help. It's knowing who to approach and what to focus on because they might have an equal amount of stress and anxiety about the situation, but they manage it very differently.

And I guess it's because Singaporeans don't see the whole spectrum or don't understand the underlying symptoms. And those are not things that you can really just experience from reading and infographics on Instagram. It requires a lot more understanding, and I think that's where the gaps are. I mean, like psychology is a subject in a lot of other countries for A-Levels and stuff. I don't know if it is here?

Si Qi

No, I don't think so.

Jolene

Or even like basic things. I know they're encouraging a lot more mindfulness.

Si Qi

Yes.

Jolene

I guess that is a good step. I think you will always have a group that will be harder to reach, and that's going to affect things. And it also applies to the migrant space. The migrant workers we've been speaking to, who are more vocal and want to talk about it, are the younger ones who are active on Instagram. They also want to have social media campaigns about migrant worker mental health. They are more tuned in to the current climate around it online, and they can see that there is a space for this conversation to take place. But the older generations, who might have been brought up a different way, who see the world in a different way, might see mental illness as something that needs to be hidden or controlled.

In the mental health context, if you know somebody who has mental health issues, it can go one of two ways. You can go, *Aiyah, better hide it, it's so shameful*, or you can find out more and become educated and then you're able to champion for it. And I think if more people are able to help their families champion for it, or champion for it within their families, that would be a more effective change than just psychoeducation.

SMALL ACTS OF KINDNESS CAN GO A LONG WAY

Si Qi

Any last words that perhaps you would like to share with people who are reading this, about mental health and about migrant workers?

Jolene

I guess I have two separate points. I think for mental health, my reminder is just that mental health is quite all-encompassing: it really does impact almost everybody in everything. You can't say it's just about mental illnesses or just about certain conditions. Anything from the stress you experience at work, to having burnout, to the slight anxiety you might have in certain situations, even if it's situational and very rare . . . all those things are included and it's something worth taking note of because it can benefit your life to have those conversations or to be more mindful of your own emotions.

I think Singapore has a very grind culture. Like people post on Instagram, *Oh look at me, I'm at my work computer at 1 a.m.* Okay, that's me too because I work late too, and these posts can be kind of funny. Until you realize you're going to get to a point where you're going to burn out. And so that culture is quite toxic, right? It's important to be able to identify and know where your own limits are, what you're feeling, and whether you can really manage it.

We want to encourage conversations about mental health in general, and a lot of these conversations are not just about specific mental illnesses. We have stress at the workplace, burnout, grief. Even grief is mental health, right? If you think about it. It's just all these different topics to start conversations. The most important thing about mental health in Singapore is just starting the conversations. There are always more insights to get, and fine, you might not agree with everything people are saying, but I don't really think there's a wrong answer because everybody takes care of themselves differently. The only wrong thing would be not taking care of yourself. And what you might think is pushing too far for yourself might be fine for somebody else, and it's about understanding yourself and your own mental health, and knowing when you need to take a step back. That's the most important.

For migrant workers, I would say that I hope that Singaporeans who read the book realize the importance of a simple hello, or a simple smile, or how far acknowledging other people can go in boosting or reminding them of their humanity. And that's a very general mental health thing as well. For anybody having a bad day, a small, nice gesture could really turn things around. I mean, you always read those super inspirational posts about how somebody who was having a bad day and wanted to commit suicide didn't because a small act reminded them of the goodness of humanity. I just think that if everybody were to approach every day with little acts that would help other people through their day, it would make Singapore a much more welcoming place. And you can't say that that doesn't improve people's mental health, even without systemic changes or any big radical policy changes. It's just a simple step that I think everybody can take, that would make mental health for everybody a lot better.

CHAPTER 12

Deepening Community Engagements through Arts and Heritage

By David Chew, Deputy Director, National Heritage Board

Heritage, like mental health, can be a double-edged sword. While David Chew warns against looking back on the past with rose-tinted lenses, he also shares how heritage can people connect back with their roots, an activity that can be therapeutic for elderly people. David reflects on how the heritage outreach programmes have been affected by COVID-19, and how the mental health and wellbeing conversation is finding its way into heritage projects and spaces.

THE NEED FOR SOCIAL CONNECTIONS

MK

Why don't you share a little bit about the work that you do?

David

I've always been working in the sphere of arts and culture. My first job was as a newspaper journalist and an arts correspondent for TODAY's paper. I covered news regarding museums, performance arts, visual arts, and I realized that it was a very exciting field to be in because for me, I think arts and culture can make a huge impact on people's lives in a very indirect way.

I started working at the NHB[79] twelve years ago with museum policy work because I wanted to understand what it takes, from a policy level, to sustain the museum and heritage ecosystem. Then I became a curator at the SAM[80], where I worked with many Singaporean contemporary artists, and I realized I especially appreciated artists whose works were first, process-based, and second, working with communities where the benefits of arts and culture were very evident. I later went back to NHB under the community outreach division, did a secondment at UNESCO to work on intangible cultural heritage, and now I'm back at NHB organizing two annual festivals a year—the Singapore HeritageFest and the Singapore Night Festival.

MK

I know that the Singapore HeritageFest this year will incorporate healthcare and mental health themes. Am I right?

---

[79] NHB: National Heritage Board

[80] SAM: Singapore Arts Museum

David

Yes. Previously, the heritage festival was largely precinct-based, so we went to certain areas such as the Tiong Bahru precinct and celebrated the precinct's rich cultural heritage and history. However, we recently decided to go on a thematic-based approach because it allows us to work with partners across the island. The theme this year is healthcare and wellbeing to celebrate the 200th anniversary of Singapore General Hospital, and also to pay tribute to our healthcare workers during this COVID-19 pandemic. We also wanted to look into not only institutional care such as hospitals, but traditional healthcare and mental health as well, especially during this COVID-19 period. In an indirect way, we are learning through COVID that people are not wired to stay at home and do the same things over and over again. I think for us, programmes for both the Heritage and Night Festival tap into that innate desire within us to know more, see more, and connect more with other people.

The festivals are a very social activity for people, even more so today than before. The Singapore HeritageFest started off as an educational event when it was first launched twenty years ago. It was meant for students and members of the public to learn more about our heritage. But over time, we've seen that the festival is a social experience, and this was before COVID. It's only natural that with COVID, there is the need for social experiences, the need to connect with other people, the need to connect with the larger things that make up our identity. Our connection to who we are, what's around us, the cultures and traditions that define us, are extremely important during these times.

MK

And this is the trend that you're observing?

David

It is, especially the social function of festivals. Any festival you look at around the world today is all about connection. It's a social activity. People don't go to festivals to learn. They will go to a museum to learn about something, but they'll go to a festival to hang out with friends.

MK

But right now, COVID is still happening. Some countries are still in lockdown, which affects social activities across the board. What are some interventions that the National Heritage Board is implementing?

David

We're going for the hybrid model this year. We're lucky that the situation in Singapore is a bit better than other places, so we can manage a hybrid model where 40 per cent of the programmes are physical. Like I said earlier, we can't dismiss that there is a desire among people to meet and connect with other like-minded individuals physically. In fact, it's crucial to our mental health and wellbeing to reset our system and connect with the world at large. Even for myself, I'm still working from home, and I do feel that it's not mentally sustainable. Especially during the Circuit Breaker[81] period when we couldn't meet one another. That social isolation was not healthy.

Even when we held online programmes, let's say on a social platform like Facebook, you can see which of your friends were tuning into the same programme and who was commenting or liking certain things. There was a social element to these digital programmes, and it certainly changed the nature of the experience and the public receptiveness to the programmes.

---

[81] Circuit Breaker refers to the three month nationwide lockdown in Singapore to curb the spread of COVID-19

CAN ARTS FESTIVALS BE MORE THAN JUST A ONE-OFF EXPERIENCE?

MK

How do you think programmes can be developed in such a way that it fosters deeper connection with people besides just hanging out together as a social activity?

David

This is definitely something I'm very concerned about because people come, they attend a nice programme, they *lah lah lah sing song hold hand*, but what happens after that? Do you wait another 11 months for the next festival to come around? No, right? What deeper levels of engagement can we create? That's why we've taken a longer time to craft and conceptualize the programmes this year, because we want a deeper level of engagement with the festival-goers. And we're finding out that this takes a lot more resources and time to plan for.

I'll give you an example. One of the programmes that I really love is with an artist called Lin Shiyun from Tak Takut Kids Club. She works with the underprivileged youth and children in Boon Lay to better understand the situations they are in, and to try and foster better relationships in the community. She proposed a programme where these kids and youths interview their caregivers, ailing grandparents, or single parents, and create an exhibition on the food they eat at home. *How are you creatively reinterpreting your family culinary heritage, given the circumstances?* Through this process, not only do the kids understand where their caregivers are coming from, the family's financial constraints, but it also gives the caregivers a creative opportunity to evolve and change the way they cook and the way they show their love and care for the kids. This entire process is documented and produced by the kids themselves. When members of the public visit this exhibition, the kids will be there to give a tour from their perspective, in their own words. In the second half of the programme, visitors will leave the exhibition space to visit hawker centres in Boon Lay to observe how, for example, the different hawker stalls do reflect the types of communities living there. After the entire programme, you also get to sit down and have coffee with Shiyun herself who brings out some of the issues encountered during the tour, for festival-goers to discuss with one another—

MK

Dialogues!

David

Yeah, where everybody shares their thoughts. We want people to come, experience something deeper, and even follow up with a call to action if they want to, such as volunteering with the community. It's the first time we're doing this, but I think that festival programmes have that opportunity to definitely engage on a much deeper level.

A REFLECTION ON HERITAGE AND MENTAL HEALTH

MK

Anything else you want to add regarding mental health?

David

It's more of a reflection on heritage and mental health. Heritage can also be a double-edged sword. When we talk about heritage, there is a risk that nostalgia becomes the focus of the conversation. Sometimes it's not helpful to look back on the past with rose-tinted lenses. On the one hand, it's really important to remember our heritage and who we are, but there is a fine line between that and nostalgia.

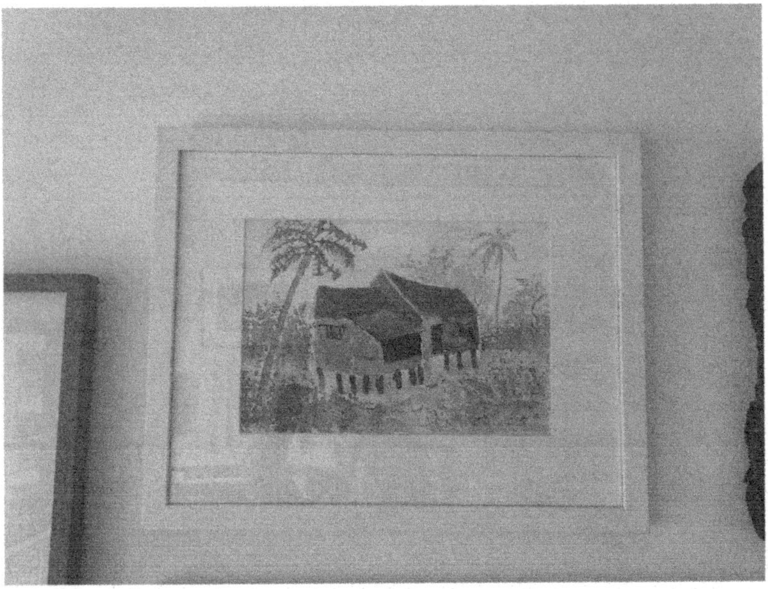

I mean to me, I think in terms of mental health and sometimes recovery as well, that's very important. One of the paintings about the kampong house right—

[David points to a painting on the wall]

It was something that was given to me after I gave a talk for the Tsao Foundation. The foundation champions active ageing, and uses heritage, among other methods, to engage their seniors and get them to remember their past and where they came from. This is done especially with seniors with dementia, for example, which is how this painting came about—a grandmother with dementia, with help and therapy, remembering her childhood time in the kampong. I think on one level, it can be very therapeutic for seniors to be able to revisit their childhood and their heritage. So this painting, while rather unassuming, has come to mean a lot to me, and constantly reminds me as I do my work in heritage, on its power to everyday people.

CHAPTER 13

Feeling the Rhythm and Dynamics of Your Inner World

By Calvin Eng, President, Association for Music Therapy in Singapore

Music therapy is one of the creative mental healthcare treatment modalities, and it is especially useful for individuals who have difficulties verbalizing their emotions. Calvin Eng breaks down the process of a music therapy session, and the ways a music therapist can help the client to express emotions and develop coping mechanisms in their everyday life. Calvin also shares his personal experience being a caregiver for his late father, and how he relates to the stress and anxiety caregivers face.

INTRODUCING MUSIC THERAPY

Si Qi

All right, so first question. Tell me more about yourself and why you decided to go into the mental health space.

Calvin

My name is Calvin, and I am a board-certified music therapist. I got back to Singapore in 2017 and have been working in the special education setting with individuals on the Autism Spectrum and individuals with Multiple Disabilities. For me, it has always been beyond the art of music, but also the science of music. I guess I have always been interested in understanding how music could be used to support the wellness of an individual and how individuals can access music to find strategies to support their wellbeing.

Si Qi

Is there any reason you are particularly interested in the disability community?

Calvin

Growing up, I had the opportunity to volunteer with my parents in the community and the chance to live overseas for quite a few years during my teenage years. I left Singapore when I was fourteen to Vietnam and Indonesia after, and I had the opportunity to volunteer in the local communities. During my time there, I had many interactions with different people from various backgrounds, including persons with special needs, and that allowed me to understand, and more importantly, know that they are just differently abled, just like how we are different. It's always about understanding other people and not putting their disabilities first. That has always been very natural for me to want to be part of this community, and I guess with the gift that I have received in music, I want to do something more with it!

Si Qi

What was your musical training? Was it piano or—

Calvin

My musical journey started very late. I started music when I was living in Vietnam! Before that, I had never actually been interested in music! I've always been passionate about musical theatre, but the whole time in Singapore—I still remember when I was in school, in Drama CCA[82], there was this thing going on between the Drama CCA and Band CCA folks—I would always annoy the band people and proclaim that I would never play an instrument, but I guess the joke is on me now. Because when I was fifteen, I actually heard the tenor saxophone in a jazz band that was playing, and I was captured by the sound of the saxophone. It was so beautiful that I asked my teacher if I could try the instrument. A week later, there was an opportunity for me to try the alto saxophone and the rest is history. I started learning music from the saxophone. I did not have piano or any other instrumental background, and my music theory was really bad. I mean, I'm not saying it's any better now . . . (#kiddingjustkidding).

[laughter]

Calvin

But yeah, everything started from the saxophone.

Si Qi

Okay, so tell me more about what music therapy is.

---

[82] CCA: Co-curricular activities

Calvin

Simply put, music therapy is about using the elements of music to achieve non-musical outcomes, facilitated by an accredited music therapist. Non-musical outcomes may include social goals, communication goals, behavioural goals, cognitive goals, and sometimes even pre-academic goals. Basically, as an accredited music therapist, I would use the elements of music, which can include melody, rhythm, harmony, dynamics and instrumentation, to support the client in achieving these non-musical outcomes.

Si Qi

In the context of mental health though, what does that translate into?

Calvin

Music therapy in mental health is extremely exciting. It may provide opportunities for an individual to express themselves musically. And what that means is sometimes, a person may not be ready to talk or verbally express, and that is okay. If a person wants to express his or her feelings, talking isn't the only way. There can be other ways to express him or herself, and music is one of those avenues.

As a music therapist, I may be able to facilitate this conversation by using the guitar, piano, or even the saxophone with the client that I'm working with. I could start by presenting my client with a choice of instrument, or if they don't want to play, perhaps they may want to use their voice to hum, or sing, or just prefer to be silent. That's okay too.

But for example, if the client chooses the drums, I will use a chordal instrument to complement their playing. As we start playing, I will also be listening and assessing: *How are they playing?* If they're playing the drums, are they playing very loud, very soft or very slow? I will imitate or follow my client musically, to acknowledge that I'm hearing what they're playing. And from there we can proceed to more playing, and I will use the moments to further assess. *Is my client ready to talk about the musical experience?* We don't have to talk about anything else. Perhaps I could ask, *Did you enjoy the jam? What did you like about it?* I might also affirm to my client, *I really like that we were listening to each other when we were playing, like when I was playing really fast, you were following me by playing the drums really fast and that's really cool!* And from there, we can build a relationship. Building trust in a therapeutic relationship is very important because we want to ensure that it's a safe environment for our client to be in, and to also know, *Hey, it's okay to share, but if you're not ready, know that I'm here to walk with you on this journey.*

Si Qi

There's something I don't quite understand. How do you kind of transition from conversations about the jamming session to whatever mental health struggle that they're going through?

Calvin

Great question! So sometimes it may not be as direct where we move straight from one conversation into another, or immediately acknowledge the struggle that they are going through. But following the example that I gave earlier where we're listening to each other and imitating each other's playing, we can use those moments to progress.

There are many opportunities during musical play that we're able to go into another conversation. Perhaps even at the start, we may be playing something fast, but after that, I may go into something more reflective in my playing. And it could even be a song that I may ask my client to choose: the term used is client-preferred songs. From that, I can explore what songs they are familiar with? What songs do they want to use? I can support them by saying, *Do you want to play xxx? Do you want to sing this song? Do you want to play it with me?* What I'm describing to you is what meeting my client for the first time might be like.

When the client first comes in, there could be a mix of emotions and feelings, and without building trust, the client may not want to open up and share.

That's why I invite the client to jam with me. They can choose to play an instrument, sing, hum, or use the body for percussion. Really, I'm not talking about anything else except the music. And it could be five minutes, or ten minutes. And as we're jamming, my role as the therapist is also to assess the client's readiness. So perhaps, during the musical play, we might share moments through the music and as this happens, I will be able to assess if I got my client's trust. Next, I may present my client with the choice of what we can do next. I'm passing the ball over to them and again, it depends on what the person wants to work on. Perhaps they want to share, or if they're not ready, we could continue with a different activity.

There's also something called lyric analysis, where I'll get the client to choose a song, and we can start by either singing or just listening to the song. We can then print or read the lyrics together. *What is the song about?* It could be something that matches his or her mood, and that's a starting point. *Why did you choose this song? What does this song mean to you?* And perhaps this song reminds the client of an experience, or a particular line in the chorus may be quite personal to them, and it triggers a memory or emotion. Once identified, we can proceed to a sharing, if the client is ready, followed by the next activity or intervention, where I may suggest, *Have you ever written a song? Do you want to write a song together?* My role as a music therapist is to, for example, come up with the chords, melody and the musical structure, but it is important to empower my client to take the lead and make these decisions first.

Perhaps I'll play a few things. Maybe I'll play some major chords and some minor chords. *Do you prefer this or that?* I'll pass the ball back to the client to make the decisions. Okay, *ba dum dum dum dum du you prefer this or dun dun dun dun*? Do you want me to play more rhythmic or arpeggiated chords?

Then, we can talk about the structure of the music. *Do you prefer to just do a chorus the whole way or do you want to do a verse and a chorus and a verse?* And my direction as the therapist is to facilitate. As we write the song, the verse could be about the struggles that they are facing and the chorus could be about the strategies that the client wants to work on, and can refer to when on their own. Towards the end of our sessions, we can even record the song or invite their friends over to share the song, depending on what the client wants to do. What I just described to you is a very brief example of what I might do. But I hope this can paint a picture of what a session might look like and how music therapy intervention can be facilitated at different stages to bring the client through different phases.

Si Qi

So, there's a lot of emotional connection and release as well.

Calvin

Oh, definitely. I mean it depends again on what goals we are working on. The example I gave could be a client who is facing a very difficult point in their life, and who is wanting to identify strategies to support him or herself, through the music therapy session.

Si Qi

Yeah, because I can relate to what you said about drumming fast and slow depending on the flow. I can see how that emotional flow works in a session, as the client goes along and gets more comfortable, and begin showing more of what they're really feeling.

Calvin

Yes, correct. There is reflective playing and listening. I could introduce the idea of a drum circle as well. Perhaps when the client is angry . . .

Si Qi

Oh, that's so nice!

Calvin

The client may be filled with anger and may not want to talk about it . . . That's okay! Let's play the drums! *Just whaaaack whack whack whack whack whack whack!* And it's okay, it does not have to be musical or rhythmic. I'll get my drums also and match my client's playing. And while drumming, I might say something like, *Do you want to scream or shout or say anything?* As a way for my client to release verbally too.

It's a lot of matching the client's present state. You have to assess what's going on and understand the client. If the client is angry, the client may not want to talk about strategies now and want to vent instead, so let's vent! Once I can meet my client where they are at, we can cool down together and work towards leaving the session in a better state.

MISCONCEPTIONS ABOUT MUSIC THERAPY

Si Qi

Does a person need to have a music background to attend a music therapy session?

Calvin

That's a brilliant question. The answer is you do not need any musical skills to participate in music therapy. That is one misconception of music therapy—that you need to have musical training. The music therapist definitely does because we're facilitating. As long as the individual is open to exploring music and being part of the experience, they can participate in music therapy.

I frequently share that we have to allow the therapeutic process to happen *in its own time*. When that person is ready to be part of the experience, then they will come, and we will be here to support them.

WHEN IS THE RIGHT TIME TO SEEK HELP?

Si Qi

What are some of the mental health stigmas that you see in your profession that you think need to be addressed?

Calvin

Personally, it will be the stigma a caregiver faces, or the associative stigma. Associative stigma is an extension of stigma towards those who care for the client, typically a family member. Hence, caregiver support and respite are just as important. Not just caregivers for persons with mental health conditions. I believe that everyone will be a caregiver at some point in their lives, be it for their parents, spouse, siblings, or kids. Caregiver stress is real.

I believe that community support is important. Because once we have a community that is understanding, that does not judge a person with a mental health condition or disability, but exemplifies a mindset towards being open, learning, and understanding how they might be able to support, we can go a long way.

Si Qi

Well, maybe we could think about it this way. Why do you think people don't step forward to seek help?

Calvin

How about this, let me share a personal experience. I lost my dad two months ago to cancer. It was very sudden.

When his cancer was detected, we became caregivers overnight because it started when he suddenly suffered a seizure at home. After being sent to the hospital, we found that he had a tumour in the brain. Since the day we knew about the tumour to the day we learnt it was cancerous, all within two months, we had to make frequent travels to the hospital and be on high alert when dad was at home, as we had to support his mobility and activities of daily living. The medicine he had to take also affected his thinking and executive functioning, and speech to a certain extent. All this was a big change for the family.

Life changed very suddenly in just a couple of days. Even for me, there was this fear that something's going to happen at night, and I would leave the door open when I slept so I could hear if everything was okay. That was a really stressful time. As I reflect on all of this, I believe sometimes the reality is not that caregivers don't want to reach out, but because there are so many other things happening and so much information out there, which may be overwhelming at that time, how do we even start to reach out? And that fear of burdening other people and putting our own problems on to them is very real as well. With that, I believe it is very important to remember that family, friends and community support is key, because being told, *Hey I'm available, I am here. If you want to, just call me. If not, I wouldn't be WhatsApp-ing you every five minutes to ask if you're okay* . . . that would help a lot too because I would know that I have people to go to when I'm ready to reach out.

Si Qi

I think especially for caregivers, the idea that *I'm caring for someone and therefore their needs are above mine* is very common. With the number of things they need to take care of, their personal needs get pushed all the way down.

Calvin

Yeah. Sometimes it's so important, but it's the individual's choice to know that *I have all these strategies or resources*, and *when I really need help, I know I can call on help* in his or her own time. Because I think caregiving is very much a personal journey too. There can always be so much support and strategies but knowing how to use them at the right time is important.

Si Qi

The right time . . .

Calvin

Mm.

Si Qi

When's the right time?

Calvin

Exactly, and only that person would know.

Si Qi

Yeah.

Calvin

There are moments when you can intervene to talk about the issue to find strategies, like in the earlier example I gave about the music therapy session. When the person who comes in is ready to begin their journey, then that's my moment as a therapist to work together on some strategies. And my hope is that when that client leaves the session, if over the week they find themselves in a low state, they can say, *Oh wait, I recorded a song during my music therapy session. Let me use it or play it now and work on the strategies I came up with.*

Si Qi

I think that on the topic of stigma, the self also plays a big role. We think about external stigma or societal stigma, but then the self also plays a part in magnifying the stigmas or creating another layer.

Calvin

Correct. This is my personal opinion, and I would like to acknowledge that others may have a different viewpoint, and that is okay, but I think it's just as important for the self to first be ready to embark on the journey.

WHERE TO START WITH YOUR MENTAL HEALTH?

Si Qi

I think the tricky part about addressing stigma is sometimes it's not the external statement but the internal stigma that we have, the things that we tell ourselves that prevent us from feeling like we can or that we deserve help. What do you think are the ways that the self, or any individual can step forward to catalyse that change?

Calvin

In my personal opinion, it's important to start having conversations. When you're ready, start having conversations with like-minded individuals. It could be family, but sometimes it may be difficult to talk to family or even friends, so that's where you can turn to groups out there. Find a group and just start exploring some of these ideas to reduce some of this self-perceived stigma. Know that you are not alone, know that there is a community of support.

I think the challenge is where to find support. For many of us who are in the sector, we already know where to search or start from. And so that's why it's very important as a community or as professionals to check in with the community to understand and see how people are accessing these resources. When they really need support, is it easy? Is it just a phone call away? The challenge, I think, is knowing how to access the appropriate resources when the amount of information out there can be very overwhelming.

Si Qi

Yeah, and you don't know which to start with right? Like which therapist should I go to—

Calvin

Not even therapy services, but many other things for example—who do I talk to first? Where do I start?

Si Qi

Do I talk to someone or, what?

Calvin

Yeah, so that's a challenge. And there's no one way but I think it is so important for everyone in the community to be equipped with the knowledge to demonstrate empathy. For example, it would be so amazing if one day, any member of society could direct you to the right place to say *hey there is this resource.*

It's important to focus on society and the community, for everyone to be equipped with the ability to just listen and be present for someone else. For everyone to support each other emotionally and perhaps not always be looking for a solution. Sometimes, people just want to talk and be heard.

Si Qi

It's about finding a starting point to kickstart all of this which I think is really hard.

Calvin

It is. It is difficult, but I think if everyone in the community knows how to listen first, and refrain from commenting and passing remarks, that might go a long way.

Si Qi

I think something we could start thinking about is what mental health or mental wellness is. Sometimes you go through life and you face struggles, but it's not like you're depressed. It's not like you're suffering from some crippling anxiety, so we tend to assume we're fine mentally. You know this idea of mental wellness, maybe it's not really there in society yet—

Calvin

Yeah, and I think it doesn't need to be there actually. For me, I think if it becomes a way of life, how we work with each other, how we talk, how we support each other, I don't think we ever need to think about it that way. Because then we become a very supportive society. To know that it's okay to fail, it's okay to make mistakes, and if I mess up, that's okay. We laugh about it and if I need some help, I can always speak to a person without the fear of being judged. If we can create a nurturing space, society, and environment, I don't think we ever need to worry so much.

Si Qi

Right, I can get where you're coming from. I guess right now it's the opposite, where we're averse to failure and negative things happening, and we can't talk about it. There's a lot of suppressed emotions. And if we can express ourselves freely, then mental wellness is always around us.

Calvin

Our journey can be very personal. There will be moments we feel alone but know that there is a community of support who will walk with you.

CHAPTER 14

Making Mental Health Less Intimidating

By Yoko Choi and Roshni Bhatia, Registered Art Therapists, Art Educators, Artists and Co-Founders of FoundSpace

Yoko Choi and Roshni Bhatia noticed that there was a gap in supporting people's needs as they worked in different settings. Beyond social services such as hospital or psychiatric settings, what other spaces can people go to for help that are less intimidating? Art offers an alternative avenue and space for conversations about mental health and wellbeing, and it gives people the opportunity to consider seeking help for the challenges they are facing. Yoko and Roshni discuss how art and mental health can help to overcome the barriers to help-seeking.

CREATING FOUNDSPACE

MK

Why don't you both share with me a little bit about yourselves and what FoundSpace does as a collective of art therapists?

Roshni

I am an artist and an art therapist. Our work at FoundSpace constantly seeks new opportunities to bring therapeutic art practices into public spaces, institutions, and community settings through an experiential approach. Although we are all art therapists, we come from diverse backgrounds, bringing our own expertise to collaborate in curating as well as facilitating programmes. We have been quite active with the youth and elderly this past year.

Personally, my art practice explores a spectrum of mediums from new media arts to traditional ones like drawing. As an art therapist, I currently have my private practice and am also involved in various community-based projects. During my training in Singapore, I worked in a children's home and a girls' home with clients who have had multiple traumatic experiences in their past.

Yoko

Roshni and I co-founded FoundSpace in 2019. It is a common place where we found each other wandering about in the unknown and incubating ideas with shared visions and creative spirits. It's like we 'found' our creative souls together, and we're continuing to walk with them. We wish to create a safe and creative space for people to find solace and a sense of self through art. At FoundSpace, we hope to re-ignite human connection to the material environment and enhance our sense of wellbeing through a very tactile and hands-on approach. Through advocacy and experiential outreach, our team works toward our larger goal of bringing the therapeutic benefits of arts to all. We have two more like-minded art therapists, Shu Lian and Xu Ning, spicing up the collective with more creative sparks and possibilities.

Similar to Roshni, I am also an art therapist and a visual artist. Currently, I work as an art therapist in a few organizations, supporting adults with mental conditions and intellectual disabilities, children and families who experience trauma, and the general public with self-care. I also teach and provide mentorship in fine art to adolescents and adults with special needs.

AN ALTERNATIVE AVENUE FOR MENTAL SUPPORT

Si Qi

I guess the thing is that we all have a childhood, and we all therefore have something that happened that continues to affect us. So mental health really is something that is for everyone. I think sometimes the problem with mental health is that people tend to put off getting help until the very last moment when they feel seriously terrible, then they'll think, *Okay, maybe I should see someone,* or *maybe I need some kind of help.* What do you think is one way we can encourage people to seek help earlier and not later?

Roshni

That is one of the reasons FoundSpace has been working on creating and appreciating art as a form of healing in itself. The effects of these are not limited to people who have experienced trauma or stressful life events. It also helps maintain a sense of wellbeing in everyday life. Making art allows us to focus, raise self-awareness, and connect with our bodies as well as our emotional needs. With sustained practice, it helps the body and mind relax, release, and rejuvenate; it helps a person grow with more clarity and peace.

We felt there was a need to make this practice more accessible to people to improve their mental wellbeing, and for those uncomfortable with seeking help, they can also benefit from the healing power of art.

We all work in different settings, and we felt that there's a gap in supporting people's needs beyond the available social services such as hospitals or psychiatric settings. So, we thought, *what if we bring the benefits of art or art therapy to a place or space where people feel comfortable to go and gain some sort of mental support through art?*

After working with Yoko on a few participatory art projects, we both felt that the audience engaged well with interpersonal dialogues and interactive experiences with the arts. Many shared about wanting to talk to someone but not going for therapy because they felt that they did not have any issues. There's clearly a need for these people, who want to come to these alternative spaces, to just *talk* about their experiences. Perhaps it's more experiential and non-threatening.

I think once people have experienced art as a form of mental health support and gained more awareness about mental wellbeing in an alternative avenue or space, they get more comfortable with the topic, and it helps them take a step further in seeking help. That's why we started approaching galleries, museums, parks, and other public spaces to engage people in therapeutic art activities and programmes. We hope to initiate or spark conversations about mental wellbeing and its relationship with art.

PARENTING: A CAREGIVING PROFESSION

MK

We know how childhood traumas play a very important role in shaping our future, our character, our desires, and even our strengths and weaknesses. There are a lot of negative connotations and stigmas around the world. My question is: what was your experience like working with children, especially where observations of trauma and mental health are concerned?

Roshni

I think when working with children, the experience can be very diverse based on their development, and also challenging because some children can't express what happened using words.

Although the adults in their lives will know that they have experienced some kind of trauma, they're not able to actually comprehend it and verbalize it in any form, so it comes out in very different ways, like in the way they interact with their friends. For example, some of them are bullied in school, so things like the way they communicate and trust issues often come up.

Also, many times children who have experienced trauma have never experienced what a positive relationship may be like. In the beginning stages of art therapy, they come in a very cautious and uneasy manner, hesitant about why somebody, the art therapist, is being so nice to them. The questions in their minds may be: *Who are you? Should I trust you?* There's always that barrier. Trust has to be built over a long period of time.

The termination period is another part that is challenging. A therapeutic relationship will always come to an end at some point. With children, especially in trauma work, it is hard for them to let go of the relationship that they have taken so long to build, to feel safe in and to trust.

MK

Got it. Yoko, what do you think?

Yoko

I agree with Roshni. On top of that, I think because of that trust and mistrust of adult figures, they also present a lot of mess-making or boundary-testing behaviours because they have not experienced that secure attachment. To them, there's no secure base in their internal life. There's no internal resource or no good internal model, so they don't know what is good or what is bad.

The more outstanding issue is the mistrust with adult figures and the insecure base. These children don't know how to relate to people. Usually, a child develops or grows up within some sets of healthy rules that are good for their development—rules that tell them what is right or wrong, where they can stop, and where they can explore. It's a learning process together with their parental figures. But traumatic experiences usually happen with a child's caregiver, the closest people around them. It's very harmful to the child's development.

MK

Got it. We always talk about self-awareness and prevention. As parents, we should be very conscious. We should raise our kids in a certain way so that we inflict less of our unconscious projections that create different kinds of traumas on the kid. What does conscious parenting mean to you, and how does it affect the mental health of children?

Yoko

You're talking about parenting now?

[Yoko laughs]

MK

Yeah, because children spend a lot of their time with their parents, generally speaking. A lot of the traumas and experiences in our lives come from our parents because of that. So, how does conscious parenting help to eliminate situations like this? How does it help to improve the mental health of a kid?

Yoko

Let us set aside traumatic experiences like abuse or violence, because I believe normally, a parent would not exhibit those kinds of harmful behaviours. That is another topic.

MK

Yes.

Yoko

You are talking about a normal parent-child relationship, about how we can be more aware and conscious about bringing up a child with better mental wellbeing, right?

MK

Yes, correct.

Yoko

Consistency. Security is very important to a child's development in their psychological, psychosocial emotions towards another person, because starting from the first day of their lives, they build relationships with their caregivers and relate to the caregivers who can guide them in building a positive relationship. They learn what it means to have affective bonding, and they learn about love. Consistency is very important in parenting. We have to be there when they need, and the mother or the caregiver has to also pick up the subtle non-verbal cues, when the child is very young, about what they need, and then respond to the child's needs immediately or appropriately.

For example, if a child is a baby, or maybe two years old, and he wants to eat, but the mother cannot provide the meal on the table or cannot provide a nutritious meal because of her own issues, the child's needs are unmet, and the child cannot experience safety because she's in danger of dying, or she experiences that she's in danger of hunger and not being taken care of. So being very consistent and being there, present, with the child and picking up their non-verbal cues with intuition, and basically really spending time with the child to understand them is crucial to the child's development.

Roshni

In terms of caregiving, in therapy, the art therapist also acts like a partial parental figure who takes care of the client's needs. If we are not aware of ourselves and our own needs, we will not be able to care for another. I think as a parent, only when we have that consistency in our own self-care, and we maintain an inner balance, can we provide that kind of attention and care for another.

Yoko

Very important. If parents only look at the child and only cater to the child's needs and forget about their own emotional needs, then they may project their own emotions on to the child unconsciously.

CHALLENGES IN SEEKING HELP AND FINDING THE RIGHT VOCABULARY

MK

What do you think stops people from seeking help?

Yoko

There could be many reasons. One reason could be that people think it is costly. Another reason could be that people think it's not timely. They think that mental health or wellbeing is not a top priority. Some might be sceptical about the effectiveness of support or help, and whether it can be measured. People may also think, *Can it really help me? Is it scientific?* Usually, mental wellbeing is also associated with other physiological or biological symptoms like headache, dizziness, nausea, insomnia, etc. People might think, *Maybe I should go for other treatments that suppress the symptoms.* I have met people who have been clinically diagnosed with depression. Just because the roots of their mental issues are hard to identify, instead of spending time and trying to look at the *root* itself, they would rather procrastinate seeking help or take some medication that can suppress the symptoms so that they can continue to function in life. Maybe they can cope for some time. Maybe they would just get more reliant on medication. Or maybe what deters people from seeking help is that they just cannot express themselves.

MK

Cannot express?

Yoko

Some people choose to avoid talking about their mental health challenges and isolate themselves because their experience is just too overwhelming and painful to deal with. Some people are unaware that they are already at the edge and that they need to seek help. They don't know how to express themselves. Even though they may have an idea of what the problem is about, it's very hard to express in words, so finding the right—

MK

Language—

Yoko

Channel—

MK

Yeah, the correct word is channel.

Yoko

Finding the right channel or modality to express could be challenging. It depends on how much and how available social resources or mental health support are. Some people just don't have enough information on where to seek help and the various channels out there. For instance, expressive or creative arts therapy is a form of mental health support, and is provided by various organizations, settings, and practices.

Roshni

I, too, sometimes feel stuck in the same way. It's so much easier for me to reach out to younger people than parents, honestly, because they are more open to these conversations. Having open conversations allows people to express themselves instead of us imposing our views on them. In our cultures, we often treat children like adults, telling them to be strong. However, it's always important to give them enough space to express their experiences, even if it might take a longer time and more patience.

Si Qi

Yeah, that's very true, because I can totally relate to you about feeling a bit stuck. How do we get people to be okay with this and therefore seek help? And I don't even know if 'seeking help' is the right term . . . It's really that everybody needs this, you know? It's not like you are somehow less than others, therefore you need help.

Roshni

We all need it, as you rightly said, to be our best selves. I recently heard of a case where a child was recommended to go to therapy by their family doctor, but the mother, who is quite sensitive to these matters herself, would rather have these conversations kept to herself. People often question the role of mental health professionals. What does a therapist do? How is it different from a parent or friend who is able to provide emotional support?

It's important for everyone to understand that an art therapist is a certified mental health professional who is knowledgeable about mental health issues, who is trained to apply psychological theories and principles in guiding a client towards the targeted therapeutic goals. The therapist holds a safe space for the client to grow and heal. They are not part of the family system or social circle of the client. The therapeutic space provided by the therapist is one where you don't need to worry and just be yourself, as it is kept confidential and private.

Sometimes, we prefer not to talk about our mental health. *Why should I trouble or burden my friend or my mum or my dad with my problems? I should learn to deal with it.* This may in itself impose a lot of pressure on ourselves.

Si Qi

Sometimes, they are the problem.

Roshni

Yeah!

Si Qi

So then how do you go to them and say, *Hey, I have a problem with you?*

Yoko

I believe you are asking: how do we communicate with our friends or loved ones if the problem comes from the issues or relationships with them? The most effective—and perhaps often neglected—way to communicate is through non-verbal channels first. We can first connect our emotions with the body before we act or think. For example, if a conflict is right in front of two people, they need to register their bodily emotions first. *Is the body feeling tense? How are the breathing and heartbeat, or even the facial expressions?* These non-verbal messages are communicated between them even before they speak, and will continue to influence the quality of the communication. We need to breathe and calm our body so that it gives our mind the space to reflect and respond to the other person. We can first express how we feel to the other person, and at the same time, listen to the other person's feelings. We need to try to empathize with each other and hopefully, this can help us to look at the problem from a different perspective. Oftentimes, we are distressed with problems because we cannot *come out* of them. And by coming out, it means that we need to create another narrative or perspective of the problem.

Roshni

Absolutely. People tend to mirror each other. Rather than asking someone *to calm down, take a deep breath* during a heated discussion, it does wonders to calm *ourselves* down, breathe deeply *ourselves*, and then move towards co-regulation.

CHAPTER 15

Culture and Context in Mental Health

By Ronald Lay, MA, AThR, ATR-BC Artist, Art Psychotherapist, Researcher Programme Leader, MA Art Therapy, LASALLE College of the Arts

Ronald Lay has spent the last ten years working as an art therapy educator, and he shares his observations of the local mental health scene in the last decade. Notably, there are significant cultural differences between the East and the West, and while some stigmas are rooted in cultural prejudices, there are some Eastern values that also support the mental health of the community in Singapore.

HOPE IS THE DRIVING FORCE FOR RECOVERY

Ronald

I'm Canadian and completed much of my formal training in Canada. My postgraduate degree was an MA in Art Therapy, and I trained at Concordia University in Montreal. I couldn't find work in Canada as an art therapist at that time. I had 250 rejection letters even though I was highly-qualified, educated, experienced and so on. And because I believed in the power of art therapy, I tried for two positions in the US after a year and was offered both positions as an art therapist. Both happened to be in forensic populations. One was prison, one was forensic mental health. I ended up choosing forensic mental health, which meant that I worked with people who committed crimes or were accused of committing crimes and who also had a major mental illness; they carried a clinical diagnosis. Primarily, I went with that population because it was about rehabilitation, not about punishment.

I worked for the State of California as a rehabilitation therapist and art therapist. I provided art therapy to mostly older men, geriatric men, age fifty on up into the nineties, and then I also provided individual and group art therapy around the facility. The facility was considered forensic mental health because the majority of the people there—there were over 1,100 inpatients—have relationships with the forensic or legal system, meaning they either committed crimes, were charged with crimes, and were convicted; the largest population at this facility were found Not Guilty by Reason of Insanity. The other group of people were accused of committing crimes, but because of their mental illness and other reasons they couldn't go through the legal process, so they came to receive treatment with us also; this group was referred to as Incompetent to Stand Trial. I worked at this facility as an art therapist full time from 1999 to 2011, a total of twelve years.

Because I was so passionate about art therapy and what I was seeing with the clients and how the clients really responded to art and artmaking, I was providing presentations and workshops all over the world. In 2010, I came to Singapore for the inaugural international art therapy conference organized by LASALLE College of the Arts. I presented my forensic art therapy work, and shortly after that LASALLE developed an additional full-time lecturing position; I applied and was offered the position in June 2011. Since then, I've been the programme leader in the MA Art Therapy Programme here in Singapore.

California was very serious about mental health and about providing rehabilitation, about providing amazing opportunities for the mentally ill population as part of their recovery and overall mental health. The facility I came from was transitioning from a biopsychosocial model to a recovery model, which was very interesting because we lost a lot of qualified experienced staff (they left the facility), because a lot of the staff—and this makes sense from a biopsychosocial model—the staff are seen as the experts. Whereas with a recovery model, the clients are seen as a member of the treatment team. A lot of the staff at that point just couldn't get their heads around that.

What's really special about the recovery model is that hope is the driving force. So, with our recovery model, if a client was experiencing symptoms of their mental illness and maybe had delusional thoughts and saying things like, *I'm the president of the United States*, with a recovery model we had to unpack that and really think about the messages behind that. What does a president do? Well, the president is a leader, they're the spokesman for a group of people and so on. So as art therapists, we are able to tap into our creativity to really figure out what's the message behind the message and can we provide treatment or therapeutic interventions aligned to that. In a biopsychosocial or medical model, the psychiatrist or psychologist would perceive the client as being delusional and expressing symptoms of their mental illness, and maybe would have increased their medications. But with the recovery model it's about reducing their medications to a certain point and also trying not to punish but offer rehabilitation and discussion through a collaborative approach.

Fortunately, the State of California was really behind the arts so my facility was able to offer a comprehensive arts and mental health programme. This meant that professional artists came in and provided teaching in areas such as African song and dance, ceramics, mosaics, painting, and so on. But not only that, the State of California also hired creative arts therapists: music therapists, art therapists, and dance or movement therapists. When I was working there, at one point, we had twenty-one full-time art therapists, fifteen full-time music therapists, and three dance or movement therapists; we also hosted arts therapies interns. That particular facility was arts-enriched.

What was incredible was that the arts were at the core of everyone's treatment and that was fantastic because for a lot of people with mental illness, they may not have the necessary social skills to work in a group or have the verbal skills to say what's really going on. With art therapy, it didn't matter if they could talk, if they could verbalize, whatever. They were still building skill sets needed for eventual communication and so on. I worked at that facility for twelve years, and we received a lot of additional training, ongoing professional development in regard to treating others as human beings. This was a people-first approach and contributed greatly to addressing stigma in meaningful and proactive ways.

TEN YEARS OF MENTAL HEALTH IN SINGAPORE

Ronald

The first time I actually heard somebody call another person a 'schizo' was here, locally, by somebody who was a trained, qualified, and experienced mental health practitioner and that totally goes against treating somebody with respect, right? What I really want to emphasize is that when I first came to Singapore, it was shocking for me. From a people-first perspective or from a contemporary approach, terms like that are considered cringe-worthy, highly inappropriate and disrespectful. Coming from a recovery orientation, it was very difficult to see that, to hear that. This experience was at a local facility, and I was with my postgraduate art therapy students at the time. Believe me, this provided many opportunities for discussions on human rights, dignity, ethics and basic human decency.

When I came here in 2011, I also observed that you didn't really see people with mental illness in the community. You really didn't see people in wheelchairs or with other visible physical conditions out in the community either.

What I can say in my ten years being in Singapore is that there have been significant shifts in how people treat other people, access to services and so on. You'll see more and more people with mental illness out in the community. You'll even see a lot of museums and art galleries bringing people from various communities into their spaces, which is fantastic because I think there are a lot of mutual benefits to be had there. The person living with mental illness is able to get out of their homes or out of facilities and be able to interact and engage as a contributing member of society. The museums also are able to increase the audience base coming to their galleries or museums, and expand the ways people interact with the exhibits and the artworks.

Our programme, the MA in Art Therapy, has also been instrumental in initiating collaborative partnerships with the community. Having a whole range of community arts projects that are collaborative also addresses stigma in strategic ways, and this does link to mental health. I see mental health as more overarching and encompassing a person's whole being. I see mental health as being related to a person's wellness and wellbeing, which I think really links back to Asian cultures and a sense of balance, wholeness and so on.

I think there's a difference between Western and Eastern approaches to mental health. As I'm here longer, I'm learning more about what that might mean; the importance of seriously considering the local and Asian context, when you're addressing mental health issues. When I'm teaching art therapy, it is traditionally underpinned by Western theories. Now that I'm doing that in Singapore, I often wonder, how it is being translated. How is it being embraced to make sense? Well, my students are doing just that. Why? Because most of them are Asian with their own lived experience, they're providing art therapy in Asian contexts, and they're working with primarily Asian people.

Over the years, I've witnessed a significant increase in job creation related to mental health, including art therapy. On occasion, you will see job advertisements for art therapists, which is fantastic as it signals the value of this mental health modality and the significant role it plays in the lives of others. I'm pleased to see an increase in local collaborative arts projects and mental health initiatives. A really creative one that I came across a few years ago was about suicide awareness; a particular organization was giving out black band-aids as conversation starters on this typically taboo topic[83]. People would put on these black plasters

[83] Bei Yi Seow, 'A black plaster, to talk about feelings', *Straits Times*, 11 September 2011, https://www.straitstimes.com/singapore/health/a-black-plaster-to-talk-about-feelings.

and it would cause interest in what is that, why are you wearing that? And it was to think about and explore the topic of suicide, suicidal ideation as well as available support in the community.

The MA Art Therapy Programme had a project called Hospice Is[84], where we looked at the stigma around death and dying. Part of the success of this project was that we were able to creatively begin discussions around dying with dignity, having a good death. As you know locally, with the different cultures, there's different ideas, customs and traditions around death and dying. We've also had projects with WE CARE, Let's Talk About Addictions. What was extraordinary about that was that we were able to bring conversations on addictions into the open and to facilitate these through art, art-making and through an art exhibition. Art therapy, this training programme, has been at the core of some very interesting and important projects.

I've been able to take students overseas and engage them in projects since 2015; we have purposefully named these the MA Art Therapy's Art, Culture and Mental Health Overseas trip. Part of the aim is to address the mental health and wellness of the student, wherein we take a temporary time-out from Singapore and our busy routine to really enjoy the inherent pleasures of engaging in our own practice and of learning about the traditions and artmaking of other cultures. Oftentimes, we partner with a local agency, have discussions about art therapy, and we even facilitate some open art studio sessions. This offers opportunities for our students to learn more about their culture, other people's culture, and how mental illness and mental health is being addressed in the region and overseas.

---

[84] 'Hospice Is . . . ', LASALLE College of the Arts, accessed 20 May 2021, https://www.lasalle.edu.sg/community-projects/hospice.

COMMUNITY MATTERS

Si Qi

I think it's really interesting because you come from the so-called West, and for us growing up in the East or in the Asian context, I think sometimes it's a bit lost on us what it means to be Asian or what those values mean. Could you give a little bit more detail about your observations on the local context, and how perhaps our culture may result in mental health stigmas?

Ronald

From a Western perspective, when I came here, I was really concerned about ethics, about boundaries, and about who has the privilege or right to information. From a Western perspective, typically one person comes for treatment or one person visits the mental health doctor or specialist, and that information is tightly safeguarded. What I notice in Singapore is that maybe multiple family members or generations within one family will go to appointments or be with the person, and there are even discussions about the client without the client actually there. Initially, I was really challenged by that, but as I'm here in Singapore, I'm learning more about what it means to value collectivism.

[silence]

Ronald

There's a difference between individualistic and collectivist perspectives, values and ways of being. What I'm learning about the collectivist perspective or way of being is that it makes sense that different members of the family or multiple generations of the family are involved. I've also made observations about how the MA Art Therapy training is really unique. Why? Because we're not just about teaching and learning with our students. We're also heavily engaged and invested with community, as evidenced through our various arts projects, and I find that fascinating but when I sit and reflect further, it just makes sense. Because in a collectivist society, it is about community. We're not just targeting one aspect or one person, we're thinking about the bigger picture, how one person interacts with or impacts or affects other people and how the community can play an important role with that particular person.

In regard to stigma locally, I think a lot of work in the past several years has been made to—and I don't like this word—normalize. The term 'normalize', by the way, is outdated and old fashioned, but basically part of the agenda is educating the public that mental health is part of every society, every community, and in order to reduce stigma, we must somehow openly talk about mental health, develop and provide access to resources and as a compassionate society, find ways to embrace people within our communities that truly respect and uphold their dignity and humanity.

When I think of stigma in the context of something like death and dying, there are longstanding ideas as to what that is. I'm not from this culture, so I don't really understand, but I need to address that in a very sensitive manner. In the West, people are okay talking about their death, or dying, or talking about services relating to their death. There is some hesitation in talking about it, but locally, it's that much more pronounced. Regarding mental illness, when I first arrived, I noticed that the treatment options were severely lacking. Today, there's more care, attention and sensitivity to people with mental illness and the nation can't ignore it. They have to look at it. I think increasingly there have been important strides in looking at this. I think even insurance schemes are changing to provide coverage for people with mental illness and diagnosis. But a lot of work still needs to be done in having open, sustaining dialogue about what it means realistically to have a mental illness, or a mental diagnosis. It's getting there.

Also, if I can add on, in regard to hospice care, Singapore was at one point lagging behind the world. I remember I took students to a hospice in London, and they were all enthralled because that setting was purpose-built and so the nursing staff were able to wheel patients out in their beds to the garden space. Well just in a matter of years, Singapore in my humble opinion, has surpassed the rest of the world and Singapore has been able to build many settings or spaces that are seriously considered cutting-edge. I believe the world is looking to Singapore now for best practices especially in regard to hospice care and some of these other areas. I've toured some spaces locally and I think even the hallways have been deliberately enlarged with the intent for people in their beds to be wheeled out into the hallways so they can participate in groups rather than be isolated in their bed area. Mentally, it gives people a sense of significance and importance because they're not being hidden in the bedroom any more. They're being brought out into the public and I think that's so important for the person living with a condition and also for family, friends and loved ones, and also for the rest of society because visibility, I think, is a key part of all of this.

MK

This is excellent because it gives people a precise context of whatever we're talking about. It is very important because this would allow us to see the bigger scheme of things. To recognize that mental health welfare just doesn't exist in Singapore. When we talk about things without context it makes it very confusing, as though it can be applied everywhere. But the circumstances are different. The factors are different.

So, what are some of the mental health stigmas you see from the work that you do?

THIRD-PERSON PERSPECTIVE

Ronald

See the thing is, I'm not providing art therapy services per se in my current role. I'm teaching about mental health and about services from contemporary approaches, best practices and ethics. It is my students and alumni that are actually out in the field and they're the ones that are making significant impact locally: our postgraduate art therapy students provide 12,000+ hours of mental health services in Singapore on a yearly basis. This is quite profound.

Like I said, I think the bulk of my response would be my observations in the beginning when I first came here and what I heard while providing clinical supervision to students out on clinical placement.

It is important to note that the art therapy training at LASALLE College of the Arts was written in 2005 and implemented in 2006 with the first cohort. It was just a few years before that that psychiatry and psychology training programmes were established locally. Before that, psychiatrists and psychologists trained overseas, brought that training here, and somehow translated those Western theories into the Asian context. As stated earlier, there's been significant shifts in Singapore, which is great.

By the way, one of my lecturers and I, Daniel Wong, just co-edited a book, *Found Objects in Art Therapy: Materials and Process*, and a good number of chapter contributors are local. Local research about mental health is emerging, and it's really trying to look at people first.

[silence]

Si Qi

Typically, I wouldn't really insert myself into these interviews, but I think I can't help but do it because I'm part of the Asian context, I'm part of the Asian culture. But I don't represent it even though I'm part of it. It's really difficult to talk about, and that's why I have to put myself into this conversation, otherwise the context is lost.

You were talking about the community, the collectivist and the family being part of the person's life and therefore mental health. I think that's something a lot of us struggle with, at least I do. Most people value having strong community relationships, but it can become challenging for the individual if the community does not support their mental health and wellness. That hinders mental health recovery for the individual because you can't really seek help. You have to hide it. Well, if you tell anybody then people might pass remarks.

Our collectivist culture has its pros and cons for sure, but I think it is also stopping a lot of people from seeking help or even talking or thinking about mental health. It's interesting that you brought up a lot about the hesitation to talk about death and dying because that's something I can relate to. Opening up conversations about this is such a simple first step, yet it seems like a very necessary thing to do now as I'm hearing from you.

Ronald

Well yeah. And what about the longevity and the sustainability of all of that? Because it's nice to have a feel-good conversation or a feel-good project, but, then what? There's been some really good Asian literature coming out in terms of mental health, wellness and so on, and it's coming out of Hong Kong and Beijing; I've found it helpful to read about mental health by Asians.

CAET (Creative Arts in Education and Therapy) has interesting articles, and it is open access too. Their last issue featured art therapy articles from Hong Kong.

Si Qi

I'm sure it would be useful for us too because the culture can be lost on us.

Ronald

And I feel like I'm in a privileged position because as a foreigner I can come here and make observations. What I have to be careful about is saying well you're doing it wrong, it's so wonderful in the West because it's easy to compare; however, there are important differences in terms of contexts, culture and in terms of perspectives on mental health and wellness.

Singapore tends to have money for projects. It's just a matter of putting it together, promoting it, because in other parts of the world, there's little to no funding. At least in Singapore, you still have access to funding and what's amazing about Singapore is there's always a plan. Can you strategically tie your initiatives back to the plan? In this case, the mental health blueprint.

It's good, because there's that backing. Something similar in the US was the Americans with Disabilities Act. And because that's a law, when I was a therapist, I was able to say, *Well, we need this because of this law*. And so, sometimes having these laws or these agendas becomes critical to pushing or progressing ideas forward. I think amazing things are happening locally, and I only have ten years to compare and contrast that with—ten years of observations.

Si Qi

I think I want to dive a little bit deeper into culture. In America, there is the idea of the American dream. I'm interested to know more about what you think because I think in Singapore there is a Singaporean dream.

Ronald

Right, and that's fascinating in a cultural or local context.

Si Qi

Yes, and because in Singapore, there is always a plan. We go to school, we know very well there's PSLE[85], there's O Levels, A Levels, or polytechnic diploma whatever, and even after that there's BTO[86], ROM[87], and for us we grow up with all these—

Ronald

All these milestones.

Si Qi

They are clear markers of what you should achieve in life and if you don't follow through with it, it's still okay but then you realize that it's much more difficult if you don't follow this path. So that's why I think the culture of striving and the need to succeed is very prevalent in Singapore, and it causes a lot of distress for a lot of people. Maybe not to the extent of mental health, but definitely—

Ronald

Well, I think it does.

Si Qi

Well, okay. It does, right?

At least for me, I do struggle with it. Not only are stress levels extremely high, but you sometimes feel stuck because you don't know any better alternative than this path that you've been presented with. And what if you don't want to go down

---

[85] PSLE: Primary School Leaving Exams

[86] BTO: Build to Order, a real estate development scheme enacted by the Housing and Development Board (HDB), a statutory board responsible for Singapore's public housing.

[87] ROM: Registry of Marriages

this path? It's scary to think about. *What if I don't do this, what then? If I don't work in an office for the rest of my life, then what the hell do I do?*

Ronald

Well, you have a mid-life crisis.
[laughter]

Si Qi

I have a quarter-life crisis!

Ronald

Or you develop addictions, abuse your children, abuse your future partner, or self-harm.

Si Qi

Yes.

Ronald

Think about it. Maybe that's where the stigma is because it's not really calling it what it is and that might also be a cultural thing because well, the concept of face is real. I've seen it even in some of the signage. I remember a sign at the lift of a man wearing a smiling mask that was pulled off a little bit, and under the mask was his real expression and he was angry because what he was really thinking was, *Don't be smoking here.* And I thought well that's a visual of the concept of face. Like I can't really tell the person, *You're being disrespectful, don't smoke here, you're breaking the rules,* I have to be nice and smile. So, there's a softer way and that's kind of like the reality of the situation.

Si Qi

And you don't experience that in Canada or in America? Not really?

Ronald

Not to that extent, people are much more vocal overseas.

MENTAL HEALTH APPLIES TO EVERY HUMAN BEING

Ronald

Thinking through your questions again, I think access to services would be another obstacle. An obstacle or a struggle and even a concern.

Even the term is so outdated, things like de-institutionalization, normalization, I mean locally, I think the community just has to be aware. There are people who experience different challenges in life. There are people who just so happen to have a clinical diagnosis. It doesn't define who that person is. Listen to how people with a mental illness are referred to.

MK

Yeah, it's still happening.

Si Qi

Yeah, they still . . .

[Si Qi cringes]

Si Qi

Siao, the Singapore slang for crazy.

Ronald

Yeah, it's terrible. I think the best way around this is public education campaigns because it should be the person first, who happens to be living with a diagnosis of schizophrenia. Or living with symptoms of mental illness, or something like that. Reality is, we all struggle in some kind of capacity.

Si Qi

I think it's pretty interesting because you've really worked with people with illnesses back in California, right? So what does mental health look like for you? What is mental health to you?

Ronald

That's a very difficult question, honestly. It seems rather simple and straightforward, but it's rather layered and complex.

Mental health applies to every human being in the world. Mental health just means how are we existing. How are we being human beings? How are we living our lives in a way where there's a sense of balance, dignity, respect, functionality, interaction, connectivity, humanity? All of that. I think that's mental health.

Mental illness is when something happens that impedes the equilibrium of all of that. I think there are aspects of mental illness that can be debilitating. And if it's debilitating, a person needs assistance, support, maybe an intervention. Because not everybody with a mental illness needs medication. Not everybody with a mental illness is a criminal. It just so happens that with mental illness, there are certain characteristics that define different kinds of clinical diagnoses. So, there's different characteristics for schizophrenia, bipolar, depression and so on.

I do want to say that the high levels of competitiveness and the significant amount of stigma around perceptions of failure are key contributing factors to mental health and mental illness in Singapore. The competitiveness and all that is concerning because especially in the last few years, I think Singaporeans are hurting.

And I really think, that COVID has drawn everybody's attention to it, and I would be really interested to see the statistics. Have the rates of child suicides, older adult suicides and suicides in general gone up? What about crime and the different types of crime, how have the rates of these been affected by the pandemic? What about abuses, physical abuse, and so on? My guess is that the rates of each of these have gone way up.

Si Qi

You mean since COVID?

Ronald

Yes. And in a weird kind of way, COVID might be the scapegoat. It might be the opportunity for Singapore to aggressively start looking at mental health in a different kind of way.

But I really want to emphasize that it's not all doom and gloom because there are aspects around the communities that are really trying to enhance people's quality of life, mental health and wellness.

Now, when I give talks and workshops in the region, it really serves as an indicator of how and where Singapore is in terms of mental health infrastructure. In my opinion, Singapore has instituted the necessary infrastructure to address mental health, I think on all levels, because when I go to other countries in the region, mental health, including art therapy, is still considered rather boutique. It could be considered a boutique mental health discipline in Singapore. However, art therapy has found a place for itself over the several years. Jobs are being established, there is a postgraduate training programme, and a professional membership organization exists here. In Asia, Singapore is actually in a really good space.

MAKING MENTAL HEALTH PART OF EVERYDAY LIFE

MK

What do you think is needed in Singapore in terms of mental health moving forward?

Ronald

This is in process already. I think the establishment of training programmes for psychiatry, psychology, and other mental health practices, including the MA in Art Therapy, has been very important; it's also about scaffolding the infrastructure. The Institute of Mental Health has been here for almost a hundred years. It has evolved in different ways and continues to evolve. My guess is, more local research, the creation of jobs that actually pay well for mental health clinicians, and ongoing funding.

Well, I'd be curious to hear from you. What do you think is needed?

MK

I guess one of the things is for example, insurance. A lot of people have this mentality that getting help is very expensive. I beg to differ, because I know the nature of the work that therapists are doing, and people don't really see the value in it. Partly also because there's a lack of understanding about what therapy really entails and how it will work for them. So even though more and more people are talking about therapy, there's still a lack of understanding about the mechanics behind it, and as a result, people tend not to associate value with it.

Oftentimes, caregivers are not taken care of, or they're abused in different ways. Their needs are not met. No wonder why they're so exhausted and many can barely make ends meet.

Ronald

Yes, I actually just thought of something about what you just said. I think having more community dialogue is key. So, hearing from the caregivers, hearing from people with a mental illness, hearing maybe from the government, the stakeholders, hearing from them. What is needed? I think people need to acknowledge what's here and available currently. I really think just having more and more conversations. It should be a way of life. It should not be routine or mechanical. It needs to be natural. How do you make it natural?

And just taking care of all aspects of a person and all aspects of a community or a society.

Si Qi

You were talking about conversations earlier on and about the point of having a few good conversations if there's nothing good done after. But I think in Singapore, in some ways you know, when I was growing up in the 2000s, there were already some conversations about mental health, or at least on related topics like stress relief and work life balance. There have always been such conversations. These days I do feel like there is too much noise. It doesn't really lead us anywhere. I think we need to think about the quality of our conversations.

MK

Hi, how are you? *I'm okay, I'm good.*

Ronald

Have you taken your lunch or your dinner?

[laughter]

Si Qi

Mental health conversations in the public space are good, but what about in our private conversations? You still don't really hear people talking about their mental health in everyday conversations. There's this idea that *since I don't have depression, mental health is not for me.*

MK

On the flip side, there seem to be more people self-diagnosing based on what they read online.

Ronald

Seven signs of depression.

MK

Therefore, I must be depressed.

Ronald

Yes, and see, we have an assignment for our students where they have to look at a clinical diagnosis. Because a clinical diagnosis of depression is very different from a street or layman's idea of depression.

Si Qi

Street idea!

MK

That's the right word.

Ronald

Because we all get depressed, but it doesn't mean we're clinically depressed.

HONOURING THE LOCAL VOICE

Ronald

But what I was going to say too is that you know what, the longer I'm here, and the longer I'm involved in a collectivist type society, being more aware of the complexities of this culture, the more I realize that we need to look at the message behind the message when people do things. People may be addressing the mental health and wellness of others without actually stating or acknowledging that. For example, some people might be addressing mental health by encouraging others to come and do gardening with them; they're not coming out and saying, *I noticed you're depressed, you're not feeling so well, come and garden with me, you'll feel better.* Sometimes I do think cultures naturally, maybe not even consciously, address it.

And so, part of our job or part of this discussion is to just sit back and take a closer look. What are people doing to address this? And for some people it might be they're volunteering or singing with others or delivering food to people. They might not even think, *Oh wow I'm doing this to ensure that people are connected with other people.* And by connecting with people, they are contributing to the mental health and wellness of not only this person, but to the community itself.

I would encourage you to look around. Because there are unspoken ways that people are addressing mental health. And sometimes do you have to state the obvious? Do you have to put words to those actions? So that it does become part of the everyday understanding?

Seriously, there are always amazing things that happen. I mean look at the hawkers. A lot of the hawkers won't tell you what they're doing with the leftovers or what they're doing at the end of the night. Oftentimes they're wrapping up meals and giving them to people. I mean that's brilliant. In a way those are mental health practitioners because they're serving the community and again that's about being a part of this type of collectivist culture. It's about humanity.

Si Qi

That's a lot to think about . . .

Ronald

Yes, because in all seriousness, when we get stressed out and anxious and whatever, it's easy to grumble and groan about everything. But I think it's just as important to really unpack some of our everyday stuff to really appreciate what is going on in Singapore in terms of addressing mental health. I do think there are a lot of caring people that are not out to do it for recognition but are simply being human.

Maybe you have one volume of our discussion.

MK

I was thinking of that!

[laughter]

I think in the future we can have conversations like this. The reason I'm not talking too much is because I'm trying to sort out the information, and there's really a lot of food for thought within different angles to look at.

Ronald

Right. And those particular angles turn into more angles to look at.

MK

Exactly, so it's actually a macro picture. When you're talking, I'm just listening and I realize that the things that you're talking about are not micro, subjective, or subjected to context or circumstances, but things we can actually look at from a timeless point. That's where I'm at.

Ronald

By the way, LASALLE has a whole collection of books and resources on mental health, psychotherapy and art therapy. If you have spare time or if you're interested, you can always come in here because this is a public space.

Si Qi

Oh, is it?

Ronald

Yes. If you actually want to check it out, I think you have to pay an annual fee, but otherwise you can come in here; any book with a blue tape at the bottom is for art therapy.

I think it's really important to have the local perspective, the local voice. I've always known that I'm a visitor here. So, I have to be very careful that the local perspective is also honoured and prioritized. Over my ten years of being here, I also acknowledge that there tends to be a preoccupation with the West. More and more I'm seeing shifts too, to looking towards the locals, so I really want to honour that, even with the book that we just coedited. We're most excited that it's coming out of Singapore and so we're celebrating that.

MK

Thank you, that was excellent. That was really excellent. I'm not saying it at face value, it was really excellent. We are glad to have you be part of this!

CHAPTER 16

The Everyday Socioeconomic Stressors Are Not to Be Overlooked

Jamus Lim, Member of Parliament, Representative of Anchorvale (Sengkang GRC)

Jamus Lim shares his experience meeting residents through the Meet-The-People sessions. He observes that when people ask for help, they tend to talk about the proximate reasons they need help, such as with a parking ticket, without mentioning that they received a parking ticket because they were so exhausted after work that they fell asleep in the car. The everyday stressors have increased significantly since COVID-19, and he highlights that there is no shame in asking for help when you need it.

TAKING CLUES FROM THE INDIRECT CHALLENGES PEOPLE TALK ABOUT

MK

From your role as a leader—

Jamus

I don't know about leader, but certainly a representative!

MK

Okay, certainly a representative! All right. I was just wondering, as you are representing Sengkang GRC, how is the state of mental health like?

Jamus

It's no secret that Sengkang is often regarded as a relatively younger GRC. But it's not necessarily the case that there are no elderly people in Sengkang, as many elderly parents live with their children. But that being said, it is true that Sengkang skews to a relatively younger demographic. Where we see a lot of our constituents fail, especially in Anchorvale, which is the division that I represent, is from the pressure they face that comes from navigating issues related to being the sandwich generation, where we have young adults—or relatively younger adults—in the midst of trying to build their own careers, but also at the same time facing the pressures of raising children in modern Singapore, while simultaneously needing to provide care for their elderly parents. The combination of trying to balance both caregiving at the young and old end, while also trying to excel in their own careers, forms the backdrop for our constituents.

MK

Generally speaking, what are some of the mental health issues you've observed happening on the ground, especially during this pandemic?

Jamus

In Singapore, as you are well aware, people don't openly speak about mental health challenges. The way people share their specific challenges is often indirect. They talk about the pressures they face from work and the need for some kind of relief. Relief could come from different sources. If they're operating businesses, it could come in terms of having assistance from the government, to help tide over a time when they are undergoing difficult times. Then, they'll have to batten down the hatches and be lean for a moment, but nevertheless, they're in survival mode. They feel that something they've been dedicating a lot of their lives and energy to for the past few years may now be threatened because of the pandemic. So, we have people who share about such mental stresses.

We also have people who share about the need for them to have support from their parents in raising their children. That is also indirect. They come and they appeal for, say, a long-term visa for their parents. They say that they're not able to afford domestic workers and they need their parents to help with childcare duties. Having parents around for that purpose is important to them.

But it can also be the little things that introduce stress. We write a lot of appeals, for instance, for parents who say that they just want to have their children attend their nearby school. That may sound like a very mild request, but at the same time, it is important because that provides them relief from logistical concerns. Logistical concerns, meaning they're not spending time worrying about needing to travel to and from their child's school, and worrying about being late for work, so on and so forth. So, we have that element of stress as well.

Another issue that may be unique to Sengkang, which you may have also heard of, is perhaps that we have a lot of overflights from aeroplanes. Sengkang is directly on the take-off flight path for the Paya Lebar Airbase. What the planes do is they take off and bank a 180 degree before they hit Malaysian airspace. What that means is that a lot of Sengkang residents, while they're trying to work from home and manage that process of working at home, have this constant interruption which is not just for a few seconds; it can last for thirty seconds to a minute. And thirty seconds to a minute for one plane or a few planes, which often come in waves can be an interruption to your day. It happens four or five times a day, and it can be very frustrating because sometimes you are in the middle of a Zoom call, like we are right now, and it's stressful. You can imagine when you have these kinds of interruptions, it may affect your ability, or your perceived ability, to deliver on what you're doing.

What I am suggesting is that these are all triggers, and they're triggers that reflect the high-pressure situation that many Singaporeans are facing. And I haven't even gotten into talking about kind of more existential issues, like how Singaporeans feel they are not earning enough, and how the cost of living is rising. We haven't even touched on those. These are just the kind of day-to-day challenges that people face.

MK

What is the impact of these everyday stressors on the mental health of the individual?

Jamus

I think the nature of mental health in Singapore is that we don't see it as something we typically go to a doctor for. It's unlike a physical health challenge. If someone has a cold or the flu, they're comfortable going to a doctor to seek assistance. With mental health challenges, I think the majority of Singaporeans will tend to bottle it up and think that this is just something that they need to do, something that they just need to cope with.

When we were in school, we had specific milestones, right? Mid-year exam, final-year exam, so we know when these stressors come into play. But in the working world, it's not specific. The stressors that come into play are less easy to anticipate, and that in turn makes it potentially more challenging as well, because you need to adapt to these stressors as they present themselves. And that itself, the uncertainty, as you can imagine, is itself stressful.

Just one more final point, and it's not so much with regard to stressors. As I touched on earlier, most of our residents are not elderly, but we do have elderly parents who live with them. One recent example we've had is of a father, who unfortunately has a history of mental health challenges. What happened in this case is that he went into a bit of depression. That father was living with his son in their home, and when they left the father alone for a moment, the father managed to identify where the keys to the doors were, and he let himself out of the house, climbed over the balcony, and committed suicide that way. You can imagine what it would mean for the son, who has to also contend with, possibly, a sense of guilt, even if it wasn't necessarily his fault for not being around for the father during that time. This example, I think, reflects how we have these kinds of potentially unanticipated stressors on our residents, the core of which are middle-aged professionals. Obviously, things like losing their jobs during the COVID period also add to the stress that our residents face.

WHAT ARE WE REALLY CONCERNED WITH?

MK

Is it challenging for the individuals within the community to step up and actually say, *I need support, I need help?*

Jamus

To be clear, we have a very select set of people who come to our Meet-The-People sessions, in a sense that if you decide to come, you have already decided that you need help. I think that the issues are much more widespread, because we also knock on doors and talk to the residents, and they share with us their stressors and their challenges. They don't attend our Meet-The-People sessions unless, as a result of that visit, we encourage them to come so that we can assist them.

The impression I get from these people who come to our Meet-The-People sessions is that they are already actively reaching out for help. But we have a much larger, dormant group of residents who don't actually express themselves, and don't reach out for help. And I think it's also important to emphasize that even when they do reach out for help, my impression is that most Singaporeans aren't even reaching out for help specifically with the real issue that they're facing. They often reach out for proximate reasons. They're saying, *Can you help me with this appeal for a fine that I received because I had parked in a bus lane because I was too tired, I needed to nap for fifteen minutes. It was three in the morning, I'm driving Grab, and it was a downtime, so I needed some rest.* They're appealing for the fine, but of course the underlying, the more fundamental reason they're doing that is because, first, they have financial difficulties. Second, they are stressed out, since driving at night may be their second job. What they're reaching out for is only a proximate reason: *Here's a very small request, can you help me with this? Here's another small request, can you help me get my child into this childcare that is nearby or this school that is nearby?* Most Singaporeans have very modest asks, if you will, for what could be a much deeper underlying stressful condition.

CONNECTING THE TRIGGERS WITH THE FUNDAMENTAL ISSUES

MK

I think it's easier to talk about mental health today compared to ten years ago, but a lot of work still needs to be done to raise awareness for mental health and suicide prevention. What do you think we need to do to support people better?

Jamus

Something I touched on briefly earlier is that I think it's healthy to feel that it is okay to seek assistance for mental health. I think, as you said, compared to ten years ago, the stigma that mental health is something that cannot be spoken about is no longer as prevalent. At the same time, I think the average Singaporean doesn't recognize that deep, persistent stress may lead to them acting out and potentially committing suicide. There isn't that connection. Because if there's that connection, then at least they can say, *Okay, clearly I'm stressed, therefore I need relief. I need to seek some kind of medical intervention.* They just see that *I'm stressed, this is just a fact of life*, and they go about their lives in the usual way.

I had another incident. A resident that came to our Meet-The-People session was a guy who, again, has faced a bunch of stressors in life. He was a taxi driver, and he had an eye condition that was causing him to lose his vision. Now, this is someone who has only driven all his life, so you can imagine that he has no other career options, and hence it is critical that he feels that he is able to continue to drive, to feed his family, and so on. What then happened was that he was able to get some assistance, he went on to Sengkang Hospital, and they then referred him to SGH[88], to the National Eye Centre, and he had to go get some blood tests as well. What happened next was that he repeatedly called in to make the necessary appointments, but was put on hold, and was told that eventually somebody would get to him, and he waited all the way till 10.30 at night, but no one called.

After that, he came to our Meet-The-People session. He had self-medicated. He was drinking, and then he basically flew into a rage and started being very angry, banging the tables, and refused to talk to anyone other than myself. And even when he was speaking to me, he was very belligerent. But for me, what I saw was a manifestation of his stressors, which was that he had an eye condition which threatened his livelihood and his ability to feed his family. He had been repeatedly told that we have a world-class medical system, but when he had, as a Singaporean, sought assistance from that medical system, he felt that he wasn't given service, and he linked it to the fact that he wasn't rich or influential. He then saw it as a slight against him and his social standing.

So, he reacted and acted out. He acted out by taking it out on other people. In the end, we were able to rapidly contact the necessary authorities to provide him with assistance to make sure that his blood test was scheduled, and we had someone call him and so on to reassure him. But I think that episode was just symptomatic of the kind of stressors that the average middle-aged breadwinner who isn't very well to do faces, especially during COVID. They face threats to their way of life, and small triggers may end up tipping them over the edge.

---

88 SGH: Singapore General Hospital

MK

Are there any interventions you think we can begin to look into, from the individual to collective level?

Jamus

It's no secret that I feel we need to have a richer social safety net. Right now, our social safety net is not only very modest, but also very stringent. Qualification for social assistance from the Social Service Office only comes when you demonstrate that you have household incomes of something like $1,900 or $650 per capita. These are very low incomes. Yet, look at the lengths that we make people go through to prove that they qualify. We require a lot of paperwork, and even after we grant some kind of assistance, it's almost always short-term and when it's short-term, we also require—if they wish to continue to qualify—them to demonstrate certain kinds of actions. While I'm generally in favour of making sure that people don't have a permanent dependence on the state, I believe that there is room to be more flexible with our social safety net.

I'll give you another story where it's clear that we need to exercise more flexibility. This was a mother with two or three children, and she had gone to the SSO[89] for assistance, and what happened was they told her, 'Okay, we'll give you assistance for six months or a year, but you must make sure that, first, your children go to school and second, that you then secure a job.' And she has children of varying ages—some of whom are too young to go to school. She then has this problem where she needs to confirm that her children are going to school or childcare, but what happens is when they go, she has to pick them up at certain times. And when she's unable to do so, it's generally a lot easier to

[89] SSO: Social Service Office

just not send them, to just have them at home all day. Otherwise, she has to travel with a young child on the bus to go to pick up her child, and so on.

It becomes a chicken and egg situation. How then will she subsequently demonstrate that she has looked for a job? How is she going to look for a job when she's taking care of three children at home all day? So, she was grateful for the assistance, but the assistance was short-term and contingent on her being able to fulfil these conditions, and she's like, *Well, how can I possibly fulfil these conditions? It's not like I'm sitting at home and just watching TV, you know?* She's at home providing childcare.

The system is really inflexible in that it requires all these demonstrations because we want to sieve out the one or two welfare kings or queens. And to be fair, I do see people like that as well, but then we also are not willing to accommodate the other eight people who are coming with genuine needs and are unable, for whatever reason, to better take care of themselves.

I feel that as a sufficiently wealthy society, we are in a position to actually say: look, there are some people in our society who cannot take care of themselves, no matter what. If they have some permanent disability, and they have been certified by their doctor that they are permanently unfit for work, what do we do? Are we willing to say, because of these reasons, the state will take care of them? As a society, that we will take care of them? But we haven't arrived there yet. I think we have moved towards being more willing to support these people, but we are very far from a society that is, for one of the richest countries in the world, being okay with saying that we have the resources to take care of these people and relieve them of their day-to-day stressors.

MK

There is so much to unpack in that.

Jamus

Yeah. I mean, again, we are starting to venture into a territory that goes beyond strictly speaking mental health but—

MK

But it does affect their mental health.

Jamus

Yeah. Because as I stated, the kind of mental health issues that I see are not explicit cases where people are suicidal and need some IMH[90] intervention, although we do see those as well. They're not the kinds that are easily diagnosable as *okay, this person needs mental health assistance, and we should provide that.* They're the ones who are on the edge—like the guy that I just described to you—who can be triggered. And we are not as willing as a society to acknowledge and talk about these things in a fundamental way, in a mental health way. We talk about these things on the edges—in the proximate fashions that I told you about—rather than address the fundamental pressures that Singaporeans are facing, which is making ends meet in an increasingly expensive society.

And this, of course, doesn't affect every Singaporean, right? It doesn't affect every one of my residents, or even the majority of my residents. If they are professionals, they're secure in their jobs, they're able to work from home. But then there are those that are less able to navigate the pandemic, because they have jobs that don't allow them to work from home easily. They are people that nevertheless face the stress of needing to earn money, to feed their families, and so on. They face these kinds of mental

[90] IMH: Institute of Mental Health (Singapore's only hospital dedicated to mental health)

health pressures and it's the triggers—like the few examples of people who get triggered, as I shared earlier—that are a short distance away from outright harm. Either self-harm or taking it out on others.

STRESS AND THE ABILITY TO NAVIGATE STRESS IS ON A CONTINUUM

MK

We spoke a lot about the collective and about what needs to be done on the societal level. What about individuals? What can individuals do to take more ownership and responsibility where their mental health and emotional states are concerned?

Jamus

It is about societal acknowledgement that it is okay as an individual to go to seek help for mental health challenges. I think that this is really crucial, and it does require a shift in cultural and societal attitudes towards being open to talking about mental health. As a country, we complain a lot: this was something that our Founding Father, Lee Kwan Yew himself, acknowledged. We're good at complaining, but when we complain, we complain about circumstances. We complain about individual pressures, but we're not as sensitive to connecting this to the pressures being so great that it causes people to break down and subsequently do things that we may call self-harm.

And of course, most of us can face, absorb, and deal with pressure. Some may even thrive under pressure. But there are also those who cannot, and it's important for us to recognize that such matters are best understood as falling on a continuum. The pressures people face lie on a continuum, and the ability to navigate and absorb those pressures also lie on a continuum. There's no shame in saying that *I'm on one end of the ability to adapt and I need assistance*, even if someone else may be perfectly well able to absorb and navigate that same amount of stress. Some people are comfortable with two jobs; they have no problems, they're happy, it keeps them busy, and they're fine. But there are others who feel extremely stressed holding two jobs, and we need to convey to them, *If you are feeling stressed, it's not shameful, and moreover, it is okay to seek help if you need help. There is a channel through which you can obtain assistance, and it'll be helpful if you were able to recognize that you're someone who needs help and be willing to go for this kind of assistance.*

MK

Is there anything else you would like to share with the readers of the book about mental health?

Jamus

I think very often in Asia, we say that it's a cultural thing, and so we excuse all sorts of behaviours. It's not just mental health, of course. It's all sorts of things. We say, *Oh these are culturally specific, they're not universal*, so we need to cater to our idiosyncratic situation, and I agree that to some extent, that's true. You need to be sensitive to cultural differences. But we shouldn't go so far as to sweep problems that are actually kind of biological and universal away.

If you have a mental health challenge and you struggle with these kinds of issues and suicidal thoughts, we shouldn't say, *Oh it's cultural for us to suck it up, and it's something we don't discuss, because in Asia we don't go to psychologists or psychiatrists to help us with mental health issues.* I think it's important to understand that there are these universals that go beyond cultural differences, and we need to, as a society, mature into and be willing to adapt and change, and not just say, *Oh culturally we're different and so it's okay, we don't need to worry about this.* I think that is unhealthy. I think we need to be more open. We need to, while being sensitive to cultural differences, also be open to allowing our society's mindset to evolve into something that is healthier.

MK

Got it! Thank you. That was really powerful and informative.

CHAPTER 17

Intersectionality Between Mental Health and Class Issues

By Jingzhou, Community Worker, Cassia Resettlement Team

Jingzhou's team works with low-income communities, with a community-based approach rather than a cause-based approach—providing support regardless of the issues the individual is facing. The intersection between mental health and class issues complicates the matter, as lower-income families have to deal with more stressors in life, and may not be able to afford mental health treatment. He hopes that no matter your age, religion, race or class, the mental health support you receive is still of good quality.

MORE AWARENESS, MORE NOISE, SO WHAT?

Jingzhou

What do you feel about mental health in Singapore currently?

MK

I think if I were to compare twenty years ago to what is going on right now, I'm glad that there is more attention and awareness and more noise around mental health. People are taking it more seriously compared to twenty years ago when we would literally just put it aside, even to the point where it was non-existent. You know when we face certain challenges, we tend to put them aside, telling ourselves that it's not important.

Jingzhou

So, like increased awareness and attention?

MK

Correct, but that comes with a problem because with the Internet, information is so open. Everybody is talking about it and it becomes confusing. How do we discern what is real and what is not? How do we discern if the information is accurate or not? This is one of my criticisms of the current situation, in that we have more noise, we have more eyeballs, but at the expense of quality, which is often the cycle of things we must go through.

Jingzhou

How do you feel that your work can address this concern that you have?

MK

We create art and conversations to raise awareness of mental health. But beyond that, we want to push for more forward, integrative actions towards mental health and suicide prevention. I think that there is a mismatch of expectations and a lack of understanding in Singapore about mental health, and sometimes certain policies don't necessarily benefit people when they are not receptive to any treatment or support for mental health.

For example, a lot of times when you talk about therapy, people will say it's very expensive without necessarily having any understanding or awareness of what therapy really entails and it can help them. People are too quick to make judgements and conclusions when in my personal opinion, therapy is affordable. And a possible reason people think that way is because they might not know what goes on in a therapy session. They make a lot of assumptions and, of course, when people don't see the value, everything will be expensive. And if I were to look at certain policies, one of the things that is still missing is insurance. We still don't have a very comprehensive insurance policy for mental health, that's something that's drastically missing.

Jingzhou

Before you ask me your first question, I want to respond to this by providing my opinion. I would like to push back a bit on understanding affordability in terms of the 'value' of therapy. I understand what you mean by this, but I think it's not completely fair to say that 'when people don't see the value, everything will be expensive'. Some people simply cannot afford therapy, no matter how valuable they regard it to be. However, I definitely agree with the concerns on how heightened attention and awareness and more conversations inevitably mean that a lot more information is circulated. I was just looking at some social media account and one thing I find is that there's not just an upsurge, but an explosion of mental health and therapy advice or information-type accounts on social media. Some of it could be really good, but some of it could be pretty much like what you said, outright misinformation. I was just looking at an account recently where there was a sort of disagreement between two accounts. They say they're licensed practitioners, but people actually don't understand because these practitioners come from different places and contexts. And licensing in Singapore and the US and the UK are all different. Most people don't really fully understand how it works in Singapore, even more so for other countries. No one knows exactly what those few alphabet acronyms actually mean. They just go, *Oh okay, they look pretty legit.* But even these licensed practitioners or professionals per se disagree about information on mental health, so psychoeducation can be conflicting.

The other thing that I've also learnt or felt is that it's not just about the quality of information I think—that's definitely one point you raised that I agree with—but the very fact that the quantity of the information obscures the real information, makes information accessibility more difficult. I might be looking for very specific information, but it's actually buried in one of the hundreds of websites that mostly contain general information that tell me the same thing. I don't need to read a hundred websites to tell me what the symptoms of depression are, but maybe I need to read something more specific about the difference between psychotherapy and counselling. We have a lot more information out there, but that also makes navigating that entire web of information a lot harder.

You talked briefly about policies, and we can talk the whole day about it, but I think in my work, and also being involved in the public consultation on mental healthcare with ex-NMP Anthea Ong as well as the conversations that then ensued in Parliament over Budget 2020 over mental health, what we see is a lot of verbal commitments. We hear that things will be done, and in media reports we are told that these issues are being heard and addressed. However, we know that usually everyone will be saying that they're trying to do something about it. And let's be honest, many people are indeed trying to do something about it. So, the questions to me are: how, what the process is like, whether what we commit to verbally actually translates into actions, and the outcomes that emerge from it. In other words, talking about things is an important first step, but not enough. And even when action is taken, we need to be critical and evaluate the process and outcomes emerging from it. Take for instance, the promise made by the government for a 'whole-of-government review of Singapore's mental healthcare system' in March 2020.[91] In October 2020, the government announced that a COVID-19 Mental Wellness Taskforce was convened by the Ministry of Health and the Institute of Mental Health.[92] This was different from what the government initially announced, but that's a start. It was then announced in March 2021 that 'the COVID-19 mental health task force will be transformed into an inter-agency platform to oversee mental health and wellbeing efforts beyond the pandemic'.[93] We know that this task force has identified three major areas to work on, but we do not know much more beyond

---

[91] Tessa Oh, 'Review of Singapore's mental healthcare system underway, as MPs highlight existing gaps', *Today Online*, 05 March 2020, https://www.todayonline.com/singapore/review-singapores-mental-healthcare-system-underway-mps-highlight-existing-gaps.

[92] Rei Kurohi, 'New task force to tackle mental health needs of Singaporeans amid pandemic', *The Straits Times*, 11 October 2020, https://www.straitstimes.com/singapore/health/task-force-to-tackle-mental-health-needs-amid-pandemic.

[93] Timothy Goh, 'Budget debate: Covid-19 mental health task force to look into post-pandemic needs, develop national strategy', *The Straits Times*, 05 March 2021, https://www.straitstimes.com/singapore/politics/covid-19-mental-wellness-task-force-will-look-into-post-pandemic-needs-develop.

that.[94] What is the task force's terms of reference? What are the processes they are adopting to guide their work? How are the public and the communities of people affected by mental health illnesses engaged in this process? The government shared that the task force is to be transformed by the middle of 2021, and more details will be shared when ready. For now, we can only wait to hear more.

MK

So, we don't exactly know the basis and the premise that they're operating on?

Jingzhou

I think we know some information, but a lot more is not communicated publicly. I would love it if they would publish their meeting minutes from each meeting. I'm not sure what's there to hide, and some things can certainly be redacted if required. I'm also concerned about who's sitting on these committees and task forces. The question of who is involved is very important because it relates to whether the different people on the ground will be heard. I believe that the people who are most affected and involved: frontline practitioners, caregivers, and different people with different mental health journeys, they must all have a seat at the table. And I think a seat at the table doesn't mean that people are power-hungry; I think the seat at the table signifies that the government recognizes that this is not a problem that can be dealt with by just the government alone. I don't think anyone has the intention at all to make the government feel that way, to make

[94] The discussion about the government's efforts towards preserving mental health and wellbeing amidst COVID-19 was based on the information available as of 6 April 2021 when this interview was conducted. More information has since been made available.

the state feel that they're responsible for all these things, that they have to fix all these things. No, I don't think so. But I think that's the challenge. On the one hand you say you cannot do everything, there are limits to what you can do. But on the other hand, when it's time to share information, share decision making, share power in that sense, then you go back to just being government-only and many of these people are just left out. Without a good feedback loop, our abilities to find solutions or progress to these complex issues are compromised.

I think who's on the table is very important. We've gathered an inter-ministry task force to recognize the intersectionalities that are involved, but you cannot catch the intersectionalities if you don't have a diverse group of people on the committee or the task force. And sometimes consulting people doesn't cut it. You need them to be involved in the process, to be there every meeting to hear what you're saying and say, *Maybe you know you should reconsider that.*

WE GET DEFEATED BY STIGMA WHEN WE DON'T UNDERSTAND ENOUGH

MK

Well, why don't we talk a little bit more about what you do in your work right now, so that it gives people some context?

Jingzhou

My day-to-day work today is working with members of low-income communities. Most of them reside in a rental flat which is one of the hardest welfare schemes to get into. The rental subsidies are significant, and historical statistics show that once you enter the scheme, it is not easy to get out of. Once you are a rental flat tenant, the number of people who stay in it for the long run as opposed to the number of people who stay for a while and then move out to buy a home of their own is much higher. That is the demographic of people that I work with.

But what is different about my work is that we are not specifically a cause-based organization. Some agencies are like, *I'm a mental health agency, I provide mental health support.* Some agencies focus on seniors, some focus on working with children, or low-income children. People usually choose a focus, a specific cause or a specific demographic even within the low-income community that I work with. For us, our work is not that cause-based. It is community-based, meaning that our work is not bounded by the issues you are facing, what age you are, or what ethnicity or health status you have. The work is bounded by the fact that we are one community. So, one rental flat community or another rental flat community. And within that locale, for instance, one of my teams supports one block of rental flat residents—close to maybe 400 households at Cassia. Within that locale, anything that happens, any issue the residents face is an issue that we will journey with them and support them as much as we can. I often say that I do social, community and advocacy work on a range of inter-connected issues. This includes supporting people affected by involuntary public housing relocation, housing, poverty, ageing issues. People who are ex-offenders, differently abled individuals, individuals with physical and or mental health conditions, and people who need end-of-life care and support.

MK

Got it. What are some of the mental health stigmas you've observed in the community that you work with, that therefore affects their choices and circumstances?

Jingzhou

We talked about this sort of heightened awareness and attention right?

MK

Yep.

Jingzhou

I would say that yes, it is true that over the years, there has been more awareness of mental health issues, even within low-income communities. Even among seniors, there is greater recognition that this isn't insanity. This is an illness. Like how you have physical health illness, you have mental health illnesses as well. But I would say that from my experience, if you compare the low-income community versus the rest of society, there's still a lot more work to do on that awareness front with that demographic, because the access to information, the bandwidth they have to process all this news and information, the socialization and social circles that we're in that will talk about these things, are vastly different. Hence, what I see on the ground is that a lot of people are still struggling to make sense of things related to mental health, whether it is happening to themselves, their loved ones, or their community members. And if they don't really understand what mental health is, that stigma then inevitably falls in. A big part of this stigma is when we don't have clarity, we don't have a good understanding, then we get defeated by the stigma. We don't know what it is, so we just plug in what we think we know.

MK

We think it looks like the solution.

Jingzhou

I think what is also important to me when we talk about stigma within these communities is that there's a lot of judgement. Recently, MSF[95] published a study on understanding the intergenerational

---

[95] MSF: Ministry of Social and Family Development

transmission of criminality in Singapore. The *Straits Times* article which reported on this highlighted that 'children whose parents have had criminal convictions are significantly more likely to get into trouble with the law themselves', and that this research paper aligns with international research, which found that 'crime runs in families'.[96] I think that these findings *may* be valid and factually accurate, but the way this study was reported seemed to me to invite judgement towards these families and further a stereotype and stigma. Maybe family issues, marital issues, incarceration history, interactions with the criminal justice systems, are what low-income families experience more. But I would have liked the focus to be on the intersectionality of social issues and class, rather than the focus on 'transmission' across generations or families. The latter is exactly the kind of judgement that members of the low-income communities receive on a very regular basis, and I don't think that's healthy for anyone. Hence, zooming out a little bit from mental health stigma, my point is that we must also pay attention to other stigma, judgements and stereotypes that are cast on these communities. We have to pay attention to how we frame our discussions so that they can facilitate helpful solutions with communities.

THE AFFORDABILITY VERSUS QUALITY DEBATE

MK

I don't really know the next question to ask. I understand what you're talking about. I think one of the things is, you know, people don't see the connection between things. People look at them as

[96] Theresa Tan, 'S'pore landmark study finds children of convicted offenders more likely to get into trouble with the law', *The Straits Times*, 21 March 2021, https://www.straitstimes.com/singapore/spore-landmark-study-finds-children-of-convicted-offenders-more-likely-to-get-into-trouble.

separate matters when in fact, they're all connected. Could you tell us more about that interconnection between issues?

Jingzhou

I think this is why it's very important to me and my team that our work is community-based and not cause-based. The thinking of issues in a cause-based and an issues-based manner is very tightly linked with the capitalist economic logic of division of labour and specialization. They specialize in something, know this issue very well, and they're experts in this field. In fact, most of society today still operates within this paradigm, this realm. But for us, what was important was that when we work as a community-based cause, we work with all sorts of issues. Basically, whatever that happens, we are concerned, we will listen, and we will explore ways to support them. That is actually what has given us the ability to appreciate the connection between issues.

For instance, you can see how financial stresses lead to very serious health issues. Both physical and mental health.

MK

And they are also the people who cannot afford treatments.

Jingzhou

Well, I mean this question on affordability is a debate that—

MK

It has been ongoing.

Jingzhou

And I think the big issue is that oftentimes, people cannot see the connection between affordability and quality. If you bring the conversation to any government agency or any politician or any policymaker, they would say, *Oh, affordability? Shouldn't be an issue.* I would say that I can empathize with why they make that claim because they would say that the public healthcare financing system largely doesn't particularly discriminate against whether you have a physical health or mental health issue. Meaning that today, if I walk into a hospital and I say, *I have no money to pay for hospital bills, I want to speak to a medical social worker to apply for MediFund*, they're not going to deny me the MediFund just because I have a mental health issue rather than a physical health issue. So, in that sense, they struggle to see what this entire affordability crisis is about. But oftentimes, people talk about affordability concerns because they might not be looking at entering the public healthcare system for many different reasons. Also, the concerns regarding the quality of the mental healthcare provided through this subsidized public healthcare system. If you turn to other options rather than public healthcare, then that is where the unaffordability lies. Of course, even when accessing financial assistance for public healthcare, it can be a struggle for different people too. So that is the nuance of how some people will keep saying it's very unaffordable, but then the state goes, *Yeah but, you know, we're trying to do our best! It's affordable*. I think this is the gap people are facing.

MK

How do you think we can bridge this gap?

Jingzhou

Well, I think that in Singapore, the public healthcare system is still very much the anchor of our healthcare system. I believe the statistics show that 70 per cent to 80 per cent of Singaporeans use the public healthcare system and I think that should be the focus.[97]

[97] Leslie Khoo, 'Singapore Healthcare Market-Share Analysis', Ministry of Health, February 2003, https://www.moh.gov.sg/docs/librariesprovider5/resources-statistics/information-papers/singapore_healthcare_market-share_analysis.pdf.

But you know, I can also appreciate through the parliamentary and policy work that I've done, that some of these problems are not solved with a flick of a finger or a flick of a switch. We talk about improving the quality of mental healthcare, and it's something that will take years. Five years, ten years. It means expanding the cohort size of psychologists, doctors—

MK

And also pumping in more resources into that.

Jingzhou

And it also takes time for the system to digest those resources to translate them into something. So that complication, unfortunately, means that we cannot afford to just work on one prong. You have one prong that looks like improving quality of public mental healthcare. You've got another prong that says: *Well, since you can't make the quality immediately better overnight, and we recognize that some people feel that it's more helpful for them if they don't need to rely entirely on the public healthcare system, then what can we do to make the care outside more affordable?* By that, I'm not talking about private hospitals or private mental healthcare in that sense, but I'm talking about maybe the in between. You have all these NGOs[98] and services running, but the costs are probably not very well-funded by grants. Or it could be things like if I'm going to Shan You for counselling and I gotta pay $20, $50 per session, why can't I use my MediSave then, since I am seeing licensed clinical psychologists too?

But I think a lot of this becomes white noise to the system when they don't hear from people on the ground. I think one of the things to also consider with this issue is, let's say that, for instance, I have a housing issue. I'm fairly educated, I know how to articulate, I know how to make complaints if I want to.

[98] NGO: Non-governmental organisation

So, I work with HDB[99], I work with my MPs[100], my ministers, we'll appeal and write those letters. And then that is how the system processes my feedback: *Oh yeah there are issues here, a lot of complaints about this.* But I think what is important to appreciate is that for people who are already in distress, for people who are already struggling with their mental health, that articulation and giving feedback to the system is challenging. It is not that these people are incompetent, not at all. But we must recognize that they face more difficulties in doing so and that is why more effort and attention needs to be put into reaching out to hear from them so that the system can process their feedback and improve from there.

WE DON'T HAVE TO WAIT FOR PEOPLE TO GET BURNT OUT

MK

Now, I'm not sure whether you're aware, but caregivers are oftentimes not taken care of. They spend a lot of energy taking care of another person, but they end up getting burnt out. What do you think we can start implementing from the ecosystem point of view so that people are better taken care of?

Jingzhou

This issue on caregivers, we can talk about it in many ways, but I think fundamentally, I'm sure you're familiar with the mantra that family as the first line of support is a cornerstone of Singapore's system, whether it is in healthcare or in social welfare. It's about self-reliance too. I think we suffer from some unintended consequences of this ideology. Seeking help is not

---

[99] HDB: Housing Development Board

[100] MP: Member of Parliament

easy when you are constantly told to be self-reliant. When family as the first line of support is taken to the extreme, sometimes it feels like family is the only line of available support. And I think that's what happens when you only recognize, or rather, when you elevate these ideologies to the pedestal, then all the stress will get channelled to the individuals, the family, and hence to the caregivers. Family as a broad term, but essentially caregivers. For example, two people with the same condition, same social circumstances, same health circumstances, financial circumstances, by right they should be receiving equal services, equal resources, right? But because one of them has a caregiver as a family member, then the care plan becomes very different because there's the assumption that *oh there's a family member, the family member should do this, should do that, should do all.* But the family member has their own lives to lead too. I think there's some adjustment required in the ecosystem, how service models, professionals, funding models, funding guidelines all have to make some adjustments. I'm not saying that you shouldn't rely on yourself or that families shouldn't support. I'm not saying that we don't want caregivers for people who need care. But I think if we want to think about how we can better take care of our caregivers, because we know that caregiving is a long marathon run, then we need to recognize that in that long marathon to run, people cannot be running alone from the start.

It cannot be just *as you run, I call for help, then the help comes in.* It has to be from the start, as they run, they are hand-in-hand in this, and I don't need to wait for you to burn out, to cry in desperation, or to say, *I cannot do it any more* for the help to come in. The help can already come in from the start, and that's how people can last longer. That's how people can better care for themselves and others around them.

MK

Excellent, I think this is a nice ending. Is there anything else you want to add?

THE BASELINE OF MENTAL HEALTH SUPPORT SHOULD NOT DIFFER BY CLASS

Jingzhou

I guess, let's not forget that ultimately, poverty and inequality are big issues I work on, and what I cannot get over is still the fact that the quality of care and support for someone with a mental health concern will be vastly different according to class lines. And I think people approach mental health from a lot of different angles, but one angle that I'm very concerned and invested in is on closing that class line. No matter your age, religion, race, and now I'm adding class, the kind of mental health support you should be receiving should still be of good quality. You can opt for some premium care lah, but my concern now is whether the basic standard in care differs too significantly.

One thing that I feel very strongly about is that today, if I meet someone in my community who has a mental health concern, my first port of call would be to refer them to a government-funded service that may not be well-equipped to work with these people. Sometimes I am told honestly that they are not able to manage some cases, and ultimately, they have to go to IMH. Most government-funded community mental health services are largely staffed by social workers. We do not have enough clinical psychologists and mental health nurses in these teams, and I have not heard much about psychiatrists serving in the community mental healthcare setting. Some of the social workers I meet also share about how they may not feel adequately equipped, especially if they are fresh graduates, to serve directly in community mental health services which require more specialized skills. And the truth is that many of these people that I work with, they don't have the resources to go and see a clinical psychologist somewhere else. To send people to the hospital at the first port of call is what no one would do, and no one would want to go into. We really do need to improve the quality of community mental health services.

Of course, the retort can be that there are non-government-funded community mental healthcare services as well. I fully acknowledge that some of them do a great job, but the fact that the government-funded mental healthcare in the community is struggling is perhaps a reflection of the kind of class difference that we're talking about: after all, these are the services that serve the poorest in Singapore.

A lot of it also does boil down to resourcing issues. Resourcing issues in Singapore tend not to just be about the lack of money. They tend to reflect that planning has not gone well. The resourcing issue is because we did not expect the mental healthcare landscape today when planning decades ago. It's not that Singapore cannot afford the kind of investment into mental healthcare. It's a question of whether there is a lack of political commitment to invest the necessary resources. I'm not quite sure that we've seen that kind of decisive, swift remedial action that is required to change that. Because we know that even if the rectification comes in, it still takes a few years for policies to take effect. However, we are not seeing significant expansion or significant investment into mental healthcare in Singapore. That's especially so when considering all the mental healthcare needs that will emerge from this COVID-19 pandemic, how many of us may suffer from trauma or PTSD[101], and the amount of mental health

[101] PTSD: Post Traumatic Stress Disorder

support required not just for us to cope, but also to heal from a crisis of this proportion. Globally, we know that the proportion of healthcare spent on mental healthcare remains very low out of every country's total healthcare spend, and it's not too different from Singapore. Only about 3 per cent of our healthcare budget is spent on mental health[102] and that's clearly inadequate to me. We need to do better than that.

Finally, I wish to end with a short note on trauma. As we speak today while the COVID-19 pandemic rages on, I am reminded about how communities and societies will suffer, in varying degrees, from the trauma caused by such a crisis. In Singapore, although we have relatively fewer deaths arising from COVID-19, many of us still suffered loss in different ways—loss of livelihood, loss of lifestyle, and more. I have heard stories of people who cannot grieve properly, for instance, as COVID measures affect end-of-life journeys significantly. We are all affected by COVID in different ways. Some obviously suffer more disproportionately than others, but the main point is that we are all affected. What is our response when an event of this scale affects everyone, with all the different implications related to mental health and trauma? This is similar to what I think about in my work, for instance, when an entire community gets relocated forcefully. We have to think of not only how individuals may be traumatized by the entire process or experience, but how trauma might be felt by the entire community to different degrees or manifested in different ways. In some cases, when trauma is more subtle, it can be more difficult to work through it as well, since it's less expected conventionally or less visible.

---

[102] Ministry of Health, 'Percentage of Spending on Mental Health, Diabetes and Ageing Versus Total Healthcare Spending in 2018 Against Amount Budgeted for 2019', 7 May 2019, https://www.moh.gov.sg/news-highlights/details/percentage-of-spending-on-mental-health-diabetes-and-ageing-versus-total-healthcare-spending-in-2018-against-amount-budgeted-for-2019/.

People may assume they didn't lose thousands of people to the virus, unlike this place or that, so they shouldn't experience that much trauma. This lack of recognition from not just systems, but individuals themselves, makes it more challenging to seek support or help, and could even lead to self-blame and the perpetuation of more stigma. It is on this note that I hope we pay attention to improving care systems such that we have better trauma-informed care, and that we not only recognize, but also resource and build capacity to support people through their trauma, not just on an individual level, but also on a community or societal level.

CHAPTER 18

Having Soul in Our Policies

By Dr Wan Rizal, Member of Parliament, Chairperson of Kolam Ayer (Jalan Besar GRC)

There are many stigmas in society that prevent a person from seeking help, such as from our parents, in the workplace, in school, and internal stigma as well. Dr Wan Rizal suggests that we create a mental health first aid and more mental health literacy programmes to provide early intervention for individuals with mental health conditions. As a parliamentarian, he shares that it is important that at a governmental level, we continue to scan the ground to understand the needs of the people, and tweak policies towards good.

SUPPORTING STUDENTS

MK

Dr Wan, why don't you share with me a little bit more about what you do?

Dr Wan

By profession, I'm a lecturer at the School of Sports, Health and Leisure, where my main job is to look into health research—mental health and physical health, which are just two of the pillars in the health and wellness spectrum. Many of my project teams do research with IMH[103], for instance. For myself, what I teach has something to do with psychology, but not *psychology* per se. But that's where the interest in the mental side of health comes in. Of course, now that I'm a member of parliament, I get the chance to actually bring forth issues related to mental health. So being a teacher and educator, I've been teaching for about seventeen years and I've seen so many students. I've taught primary school, secondary school, polytechnic, and of course university. I missed the ITE[104] and the JC[105] students, but I got to interact with many students, and I've seen instances where students go through nervous breakdowns and mental health issues.

Although I've never had a direct experience, I know some of my colleagues have had their students go through suicide, and this affects me as an educator. I love how students develop, and it saddens me when things go the other way. Those are my motivations. My first interaction with a suicide incident was through my NS[106] vocation. I was a Rota commander in a fire

[103] IMH: Institute of Mental Health (Singapore's only hospital dedicated to mental health)

[104] ITE: Institute of Technical Education

[105] JC: Junior College

[106] NS: National service

station and was called up for a suicide call. When I met the person, he shared a bit about why he was feeling that way, and he made me think further. Life doesn't revolve around you and there are many people who are going through difficulties all the time. It keeps you rooted, for me. So that's important. Hope that's a good introduction!

MK

Got it. There's a lot of empathy, a lot of active listening, a lot of compassion, I think, that's required.

Dr Wan

Indeed. And especially now, being an MP[107], all these traits that you mentioned get amplified because you meet people often. Sometimes they're happy, sometimes they're hiding something, but you try to listen and provide as much support as possible anyway, and that makes whatever I do now even more meaningful, I would say.

STIGMATIZATION HAPPENS ACROSS YOUR WHOLE LIFESPAN

MK

I want to ask—because you work with a lot of people on the ground on a personal level as well as at the community level—what are some of the stigmas around mental health that you've observed?

Dr Wan

At its crudest level, when someone has a mental health issue, it can be joked about. It's as simple as that. People joke, *Aiyah, you're*

[107] MP: Member of Parliament

so weak, can you have more mental strength? Can you toughen up? These are not healthy because you're pushing aside someone's problem or difficulties they face. It may seem simple, but it has a deeper impact because here you have someone who wants to share with you as a friend, and you—as a group, or a person—are pushing it down. And it's not right.

The next level is more serious, where you confide in your parents. Generally, when you look at how the older generation takes mental health issues, they take it really negatively. It's easy to label someone crazy immediately, right? *Are you crazy?* And they start to label someone very easily. Maybe it's a generational issue. They were from the generation of grit. They went through much tougher times, so maybe we can understand where they're coming from, but it's something that needs to be looked into in the current context.

I do feel that stigmatization gets worse in the workplace. When you stigmatize someone, the impact is not just about getting them to rest. You lower their workload, and it becomes part of the work plan, part of their assessment. I talked about grading also recently in parliament, about how it's not healthy for mental health, how we're always fighting for better grades at work. When someone confides in you, and they need some space, they get penalized for that. That's also something that I feel is not right.

And when we talk about school, there's pressure. I'm quite lucky. For me, having gone into the normal stream was a blessing. I managed to go through things at my own pace, and it helped me personally. And now they're removing it, right? I think that the government has done a good job trying to remove all this banding. I'm quite confident that at least we understand that grades are not everything. I think that is the important point MOE[108] is trying to push, so I am aligned with that and grateful to be part of the community that continues to discuss this.

---

[108] MOE: Ministry of Education

And we have the elderly who are also being stigmatized, right? You know the elderly. The moment they show signs of dementia or forgetfulness, people stigmatize them as gone. Stigmatization happens across your whole life span. The moment you're born, you can be stigmatized in school, by your friends, and all the way to the elderly stage. Stigmatization, like I mentioned in parliament, is a real issue, but I cannot. I'm the sort who does not believe that ranting about it will help. I thought in parliament I would put forth some strategies that would cause behavioural change in people and hopefully reduce the stigmatization. It can be as simple as wanting to seek help, but fearing that going to the doctor or getting help at the hospital will worsen the stigma against them and the people around them. We have to reduce this.

MK

What do you think is holding people back from looking for help?

Dr Wan

I look at it from two levels. One is internal. So internally, you have a set of ideals that *if I do seek help, it's wrong*—and this is based on past experiences. There's peer pressure—asking for help means people will know, and people knowing means it's shameful, right? They're so worried about that. *How does it impact me in terms of career progression? How does it impact me in terms of acceptance in the family?* Which is wrong, *totally wrong*. On the external level, it's about how they themselves maybe don't even understand that they're having mental health issues. Before I talked in parliament, I met with many people with mental health issues and they shared with me that they didn't know they had mental health issues and the reason that maybe they didn't know how to read the signs, or maybe they were lost. That's why I think it's important we have mental health literacy, so at least if you don't see it, someone who can see it can help you.

CYBERBULLYING—IT'S EVEN EASIER TO MASK PAIN AND HURT

MK

I want to ask you something. I think it was some time last year, during parliament, when you spoke about cyberbullying. I feel that this is a very important conversation that generally the public should have more because we don't know enough about it.

Dr Wan

True. I feel strongly about for cyberbullying simply because I see it happening around me quite a bit. And for students in polytechnic and university, social media is kind of like their second life, you know?

But cyberbullying aside, bullying itself is wrong! And I've always found an issue with bullying. When I was growing up, I was really skinny, I wasn't so smart, and I was susceptible to being bullied in school. And it was not easy for me. The bigger people bully the smaller ones and it seems okay to a certain level. *But it's not okay*. And now it has manifested as cyberbullying. Now, you don't see the cuts people get or the bruises people get. It's worse because you can't see this through cyberbullying. Whatever hurt someone goes through as a result of this bullying is no longer obvious. Last time when people asked me, are you being bullied? I say, *No I'm not, I'm okay*. It's the same now, right? But this okay-ness is the thing that leads to more issues. When it comes to cyberbullying, I am totally against it. I've raised it a few times in parliament and asked how we can look into this because now, cyberbullying isn't just about students in schools, but it extends to adults and the elderly. They're also affected by cyberbullying because of digitalization. These are some of the issues we must tackle. Are we nearing any form of a resolution? No. But one thing's for sure: when you have cyberbullying, people are affected, and this is something we should come down hard on. Is it easy to police? I do not know, I think—

MK

When there's an aggressor, there must also be a victim, so somebody must be suffering. And sometimes the aggressors themselves are the victims from other places. And it creates a spillover effect in different areas of their lives. At the end of the day, it's really about looking inwards into themselves.

What is causing them, really causing them to act out the way that they act? And for the people who are being bullied, what is really causing them to react the way they react? What is really stopping them from fighting for themselves or making a stand for themselves? I think there are many layers to this. It's not about who is right or who is wrong.

CREATING A MENTAL HEALTH SAFETY NET

MK

What can we do as a community to support one another to get through difficult times, difficult emotions, especially in the post pandemic lockdown that we just dealt with?

Dr Wan

First, we need to identify what the mental health issues are. How do I know that you're suffering from depression, or you're going to suffer from depression, or you're showing signs and symptoms of such behaviour? I think that must be the number one issue, because if you do not know, you'll keep on joking about it.

But if you make it a point to understand, and everyone goes through mental health literacy, you go through what I call a mental health first aid. You go through physical first aid, but do we have mental health first aid?

MK

Do we also have emotional health first aid?
[MK laughs]

Dr Wan

Exactly! Do we even have that? Because we know that if someone gets cut, that is first aid, but—

MK

What about the psychological cuts, the invisible wounds?

Dr Wan

Yeah, exactly. Do we need this? I think it's about time we asked ourselves what we need to do more. I think literacy programmes are the first level. At the very least lah, at the very least build that foundation. Mental health literacy, and a cyber wellness kind of literacy too. Right now, there are no rules in cyberspace!

MK

It's a free open space and people are just doing whatever they want. People can hide behind screens.

Dr Wan

Exactly, and they do not know what effects they have on people when they pass out such comments. Memes are funny, but we tend to forget that someone gets hurt somewhere in the process, and this is something we need to really, *seriously* look into. I also mentioned how we need to provide mental health leave. I was looking more from the student's perspective. I have students who don't want to come for certain modules, but what if they skip lessons because they are going through some mental health issues? I was hoping that if we allow them to take this leave, at the very least we know. It's a signal. Taking a one-day leave is fine, maybe you need a break, but if you take it often, it's a sign. For an educator, when do we know if our student is not doing well? Mid-terms, which is halfway through the semester? That's a bit too late. If I want to help my students, I want to help them from the start.

THE ENVIRONMENT, THE PEOPLE, AND THE LAW

Dr Wan

My PhD was on the dynamical systems theory. So dynamical systems mean that we appreciate that the world is dynamic. Everything is dynamic, and things move a lot all the time. And they're not just moving a lot all the time, they're interdependent, and that's when theories like the butterfly effect come in. And it can be as simple as the butterfly flapping its wings that causes a tsunami. Me being born in a South American country or being born in China could have two different effects on how we are shaped as a person, you know. My living conditions and environment can shape me too. Whether I'm born rich or poor, whether the environment allows me to thrive, or allows me to do things that matter.

When we look at individuals, we must understand that every individual is unique. I think this is something we tend to forget. We tend to have a cookie-cutter approach when we look at people, saying, *Oh this guy is from here, he's like that.* And that's not really true, because even at the physical level, each individual is different and unique. There are deeper issues when it comes to judging, and I always believe you should judge less and help more. I always tell everyone who's helping out, when you're working with me and working with community, you can't judge, because the moment you judge—

MK

You start running your own projections instead of listening to what the person really needs!

Dr Wan

Yeah! And you should just focus on helping people. The more we start to judge character or appearance, we affect the whole idea of doing good. But anyway, moving back to the individual—the individual is unique in their physical aspect, so what about the mental aspect? Because there are countless layers that one experiences in any emotional rollercoaster that one goes through. You never know how resilient a person is, how they'll react to certain things, and everybody reacts differently! Which brings me to my last point—where rules and policies make a difference.

I'll give you an example. There are certain rules and policies that do not promote mental health, and that would affect the whole situation altogether, right? But there are rules and laws out there that can be adapted and modified to suit different environments and individual needs to produce something beautiful. And that's where I feel my role as a parliamentarian plays a part, because we can set certain guidelines and rules in parliament and push for change. And I think this is important to understand. Wherever we go, we must always consider these three aspects. The environment, the people, and the laws. Like people say, right? *When in Rome, do what the Romans do.* And it's so true, because the laws affect them. And on our own, we should always be continuously scanning the ground from a governmental level to understand the needs of the individual, the environment, and tweak towards good. Structures are important, but it's also important to know that structures can also be modified, adapted and changed with time.

That's the beauty about, you know, us. We are a secular country, like many people say. But we have soul. Think about it. For me, I think about it all the time. Not many countries allow us to, like for example in my religion, I'm allowed to do what I want to do. I am allowed to fast and I won't get penalized for it, and everybody gets a chance to do it. And this is something I think I am fighting for all the time—to make sure that we continuously have soul in all our policies.

MK

Soul in our policies. Thank you for your time. I thought it was amazing.

CHAPTER 19

Bridging Business and Wellness Objectives

By Michael Chang, Director, Government Relations, Singapore International Chamber of Commerce

Michael Chang believes that it is of critical importance for leaders to explore ways to achieve business objectives in a manner that is not detrimental to the staff's wellbeing. He stressed that unlike achieving business revenue goals, shifting the culture and values of the organization to one that bridges business and wellness objectives often takes time and patience, and leaders cannot rush in the process of creating safe spaces for employees.

RECOGNIZING MENTAL HEALTH IN THE WORKPLACE

MK

Why don't you share with us a little bit more about what you do to give the readers more context?

Michael

I'm the Director of Government Relations at the Singapore International Chamber of Commerce (SICC). I primarily deal with the various government agencies in Singapore for the purpose of helping our member companies, which are mostly businesses. It could be about employment pass issues, it could be about economic policies, it could be about grants, it could be about new reporting guidelines as imposed by the various agencies. Anything related to helping businesses in Singapore, making things smoother for them . . . that's part of my role.

The second part of my role is looking after twelve interest groups in SICC. The interest groups are basically ground-up initiatives, where member companies who have a common interest come together to talk, discuss, share information and explore ways of improving their knowledge, skills, and business opportunities in Singapore. And of course, the interest group is a good way for them to network and meet new people outside of their own industries.

MK

Got it. In your role itself, what is the importance of mental wellness at an organizational level? Because when we talk about mental wellness, usually people would think from an individual level, but based on your role in the organization, how do you see it as a concept within the organization itself?

Michael

For me, mental wellness is equally, if not more important than physical wellness. We worry a lot about our health. We exercise, we watch what we eat, we make sure we drink water, we do this, we do that. But what many people don't understand is that the most important part of our body function comes from the brain. The mental aspect. When it comes to sports, when it comes to physical activity and exercise, many people do not realize that it is the mental toughness that is sometimes more important than your physical fitness. And it is the same in an organizational aspect as far as I'm concerned. No matter how intelligent or how good a salesperson you are, no matter how good a staff you have, if that particular individual is not mentally or physically capable of carrying out his duties, his work is going to suffer. And by extension, his teammates, and therefore his boss, his subordinates, and the entire organization, will suffer. It's like a clock. If one part of the clock fails to function, then the clock breaks down, slows down, or tells the wrong time.

MK

And as a whole, what is the consequence that you have seen based on your experience itself?

Michael

Based on my experience, the worst example I have seen is an individual breaking down in tears in the middle of the meeting, having to go for counselling, and being out of action for two and a half to three months. And at the end of the day, who suffers? And as I mentioned earlier on, the team suffers. And by extension, the entire organization gets impacted. So that's from an organizational point of view, but I think focusing on the individual point of view is worth it because nothing is more important than your wellbeing. No work, no salary, no job, is worth sabotaging your own health for, whether it's physical or mental.

MK

What do you think that many organizations out there right now can do more effectively in order to build a community or culture within their organization that really emphasizes on mental wellness?

Michael

For me, there are two portions to this. Businesses exist for a reason. Businesses exist to make money for profit. How else are they going to answer to their stakeholders and shareholders? How else are they going to pay salaries and bonuses? How else are they going to come up with services that help other companies, other sectors, and other industries? I don't dispute the importance of why businesses exist in the first place. To me, to answer your question directly, it is of critical importance for leaders to explore ways to achieve business objectives in a manner that is not detrimental to the staff's wellbeing, whether it is physical or mental. You don't overwork them, you find ways to make sure everyone has enough rest, that everyone is mentally motivated, and everyone is taken care of. You lead. You do not manage.

There are so many examples of people wearing a badge on their shoulders. Being busy is like a badge of honour. *I worked until midnight last night. I'm still replying to emails over Saturday and Sunday. I had to submit my paper, and I was doing it over the weekend at the expense of family time and downtime.* And people wear it proudly like a badge. There's no such thing as downtime, all in the name of operational excellence, of being a conscientious worker, etc. I think it is a culture that is neither healthy nor sustainable for the business, and definitely not for the individual.

Leaders have to find a way to achieve both objectives. It's not fair on the flip side for me to talk about focusing on the wellbeing of staff and individuals, and then the company goes bankrupt. I don't think that's fair.

MK

So part of it is also about managing expectations and creating values.

Michael

Certainly. Value systems. I think many large companies and organizations have what we call the core values of the organization. But how many leaders actually practice and implement internal policies to achieve these values? Do they actually have a tracking system in place? What I know is that there are many who don't. This is one area leaders need to explore in order to meet both objectives of company revenue, profits, operating excellence *vis-à-vis* the mental and physical health and wellbeing of staff.

STEPPING INTO EACH OTHER'S SHOES TO CREATE SAFE SPACES

MK

How do you think organizations out there can do better, especially in recent times when COVID has already happened? Most organizations are alternating between working from home and going back to the office.

Michael

For me, there are two parts to your question. First and foremost, I think leaders themselves are facing enormous stress and pressure from the pandemic situation. They have to deliver results, yet at the same time, they are human beings too. They also have to work from home, they also have children and aged parents who maybe got affected by COVID. Their lifestyles have to change as well. Children are no longer allowed to go to school or they have to study from home. So as far as I'm concerned, leaders are also human. They are no different from their staff. First and foremost, they need to put themselves in the shoes of their subordinates, especially those at the highest level in order to understand what the lower echelons can go through. Hopefully, they themselves have also gone through it because they are also humans, and that is the first important step.

The second part is about how we communicate with each other. It doesn't matter what level the individual is at. They can be at the lowest level or the CEO level. How do people in the organization communicate with each other? To me, that is very important to creating a safe space for honest communication, especially around difficult conversations, like, *I'm in trouble, I cannot handle it, I cannot manage it.* And like I said, it doesn't matter at what level, at what appointment he or she is, there must be a safe space created so that the individual is not penalized. The individual must not be under the impression that *I'm gonna lose my job, I'm gonna get sacked. I'm gonna get no bonus because I'm asking for help, because I'm not pulling my weight, because I'm not doing what I'm supposed to do.*

MK

Got it. Now, I want to talk a little bit more about what you just mentioned about difficult conversations. As leaders and managers out there, how can we build a safer space for their team members to actually come forward to them to have these difficult conversations that can be very controversial? Of course, like I said, as we are more open as individuals, another issue that might come is some people might choose not to take responsibility for what they're dealing with and dislodge their responsibilities to the team.

Michael

Yes. What you have asked is a million-dollar question. There can be thousands of ways a leader can try to enforce a safe environment for difficult conversations. But there are so many different factors involved. There is this quote I find very meaningful: 'People do not fake their unhappiness. People do not fake depression. People fake being well.' They fake their wellbeing. They put on a false front. They hide what they're going through no matter how difficult the times. They don't say anything, and then they pretend on the outside that they're perfectly okay.

I think it is very meaningful in that whether you are a co-worker or whether you are a leader, how do you identify individuals within your organization who are struggling if they don't tell you? And after identifying it, how do you find a correct way to approach the individual, such that the individual opens up? Even if you identify it correctly, which is difficult enough already, if you approach the person wrongly and ask the wrong question, the person may shut off even more or get defensive. The second part is how do you create company culture, like what you mentioned earlier? That has to come from the top. From the board of directors, CEO, senior management team—how do they lead by example, show, and convince people? It is not something that will happen overnight unless you have been doing it consistently over the years. So many times, leaders again, unfortunately, are objective-driven people. They are very impatient people. They want results and want to see results immediately, and expect the same from organizational change, which is wrong. You cannot rush cultural and organizational change. Mindset is the most difficult part of change, so I think as far as changing the organizational culture and mindset, start as early as possible but do not expect overnight improvement immediately. They have to be patient. The third part is avenues where individuals can find an anonymous way to raise their concerns. Such ways can be simply writing or typing things down on a piece of paper anonymously and slotting it into a box. There are many ways in which you can try to create a safe environment. Start small, think big, but you have to do it early. If it is not already in place, I think it is always a good time to start. Better late than never. In my opinion, these are the three most important things that popped into my mind.

MK

Got it. Any final words you would like to share with readers in terms of mental wellness, mental health, and emotional health?

Michael

I just want to say something that was said by a man wiser than me. It is never a shame to ask for help. It is never a shame to show weakness. In fact, it takes a lot of strength and courage to put your hand up and say I need help. I think to me, this is probably the key message I want to send out to readers because the people around you, whether your friends or family members, your bosses, HR managers . . . they can do whatever they want, they can do whatever they can, but it always takes two hands to clap. And if you're unwilling to respond, if you're not willing to open up, then it's very hard for anyone to help.

CHAPTER 20

Becoming Conscious of the Impact We Have on Each Other

By Victor Mills, Chief Executive, Singapore International Chamber of Commerce

Prioritizing profit over people, managing upwards, and getting into inner political circles are some of the issues causing organizations to excuse bullying or bad behaviour at the workplace. With over forty years of experience in the workplace, Victor Mills shares his firm conviction that organizations owe a duty of care to its employees, and the best way to do that is to co-create and co-sustain with their teams a positive workplace culture.

ENABLING A POSITIVE WORKPLACE CULTURE

MK

All right Victor, good morning! Why don't we begin this conversation with you introducing yourself to us?

Victor

I'm originally from Northern Ireland. I've been in Singapore for thirty-seven years. What brought me to Singapore originally was my job. I used to work for a bank, and in those days you had no choice over your posting, where you were posted to, what job you did, or when it happened. I was lucky that after my first posting in Hong Kong, I got my second posting in Singapore. That's how I arrived in Singapore back in early 1985. I spent thirty years in banking—ten years as a commercial banker, and twenty years as an institutional banker. My customers were other banks—central, commercial, and private banks. And then I left banking and went to the Singapore International Chamber of Commerce. I've been working for the Chamber for over nine years, and I'll complete eight years as Chief Executive in June this year.

MK

Nice, nice. In the context of mental wellness in organizations, what are some of the things you see that are important for mental wellness, from an individual level to an organizational level?

Victor

Well, mental wellness is a huge topic. People go through their lives and they may very well have multiple instances of mental ill-health because of whatever life throws at them. It could be tragic deaths, it could be heartbreak, it could be illness, it could be all sorts of things. But in terms of an organization, I really believe that the organization owes a duty of care to its employees and the best way for the organization to deliver on that is to co-create and co-sustain with their teams a positive workplace culture. And what I mean by positive workplace culture is a workplace culture where nobody is abused, bullied, discriminated against, harassed sexually or otherwise, or undermined by anybody in that organization. My contention is that each organization at the board level needs to sit down and think, *What are the values we subscribe to, and what are the behaviours that demonstrate those values we are going to expect from everybody in the organization?* And once they've gotten those ideas, they need to socialize them with their teams to make sure they haven't missed out on anything important. Once that's agreed upon, they need everybody on board to communicate it to every people manager, every supervisor, and every individual. And then they must walk the talk. Because without that, there's absolutely no credibility. Everybody in the organizations always looks for the difference between words and actions. And where there is a difference, and that difference is not addressed, then you get a dollop of cynicism and the feeling that *it's just like that* and you just have to put up with it. I genuinely believe that this is not just a nice-to-have. It is absolutely critical for sustained commercial success. Because as we all know, happy people produce happy customers, and they in turn produce happy repeat customers, and the revenue of the business is sustained.

I know a lot about this from my own personal experience in banking when—certainly in my days, and I have no reason to suspect that it's changed dramatically—there were a lot of toxic bosses who, because of their ability to manage upwards politically for themselves, managed to bully their teams on an ongoing basis and you've got every type you can think of. And because of the revenue they generated, they got away with blue murder. And that caused untold damage to many of their team members' individual health—physical as well as mental. And the only solution was to get out, to leave. And I experienced this for myself. I worked for fifteen years for one of the world's most toxic people, and I finally got out because it was going to kill me. It was absolutely going to kill me. It was unremitting, constant smiting, undermining, and bullying. And it didn't matter what I did; it was never good enough. And it didn't matter what my successes were; it was just glossed over. And it was due to that individual's own insecurity. And I've noticed that about bullies that I've come across and worked for: they are in themselves very insecure about people and their way of handling that insecurity is to basically bully other people. It makes them feel as if they've achieved something. And I think that's a real shame because it holds everybody's development up. In an ideal organization, that would never have happened because there would have been mechanisms for me to whistle-blow. The only mechanism I had was to use an employee's assistance programme and go and talk to somebody who was not involved. In other words, a professional. And that, I think, is at the crux of the issue.

Some other people have said to me that in situations where they find themselves like that, it wasn't so much the insecurity of the boss, but the complete and utter lack of self-awareness where they were completely unaware of how they dealt with others. And this whole experience was extraordinary because without me realizing, I was pushing the stress that I was experiencing down on my team. And I only stopped doing that when one of the youngest members of the team came to see me *and said, 'You know, we can't go on like this'.* And I was completely unaware of the impact I was having on others. And this is where it is absolutely essential for all of us to be very self-aware about who we are, what we're doing, what we're saying, and to be conscious of what we say and the impact that may have on other people. I was so shocked because I always thought of myself as a nice guy, that I literally took the afternoon off and went away. I went for a long walk to think about this and I could see that my colleague was right! And I vowed that day that whatever stress I was experiencing, I would not pass it down to my team and, in fact, I would find a way to get out of that situation. And I eventually did. I got out of that team. I left the toxic boss, which is what a lot of people do. And that experience was absolutely fundamental to the way I see workplace culture and how I see work as a collaboration.

And the big changes we need in our society are for business leaders to realize the impact they have on their teams and to work with their teams so that everybody learns how to self-manage. And this is a big change, because in many organizations, it's very much top-down, and employees tend to wait until they're told to do something. But what self-management demands is that organizations co-create and co-sustain a positive workplace culture with their teams and with their superiors in the organization. It also demands penalties for non-compliance so that if somebody, whether it's a boss or it's an individual, does not practice the agreed desired behaviours, the penalties for non-compliance are there, and they are enforced irrespective of seniority or revenue-generation, which are usually the get-out clauses for a lot of bad behaviour.

And this sort of financial services industry is by no means unique. In fact, since I've been doing this job, I've had lots of contacts across sectors and this type of behaviour is very common in organizations. And this is one of the reasons why I believe in the thirty-seven years I've been here, the general level of mental wellbeing has reduced significantly. And it's only now because of the pandemic, because senior folks in companies have to shoulder all the burden of, *How do we respond to this? How can we survive? How can we get ourselves out of this terrible mess?* They too were experiencing a lot of mental ill-health and were finally driven to talk about it. And suddenly mental wellbeing is now out of the closet. It's one of the silver linings of the pandemic, that people are more aware than ever before. And it's not just people like you in your work, but also people in business who are more aware than ever before, of the impact of mental health on individual careers and on corporate success. So that's a real positive change. What I'm hoping is that that will push people to realize that if you want good mental health in the workforce, you really need to enable a positive workplace culture and the ancillary benefit of that is that it will resolve all the other problems that exist in the commercial and corporate world. The issues of fair hire or unfair hire. The issues of people being passed over for a promotion. If you have a positive workplace culture, there are mechanisms, policies and procedures to prevent that type of thing because that kind of behaviour is inconsistent with the values of the business and the behaviours that demonstrate those values.

BUILDING CONSCIOUS SELF-AWARENESS IN ORGANIZATIONS

MK

Nice. That's a lot of wisdom. I was just wondering . . . in your opinion, how can we develop more consciousness and self-awareness in organizations as a whole? For example, instead of just concluding that bosses and certain people in the team as toxic, what are some of the red flags that people can be aware of so that they can notice these issues sooner? And if people are aware of these red flags, how can they communicate more effectively to address these things? Because like what you said, some people are just not aware at all, of how their actions have a cause and effect on their teams and the business.

Victor

It's a very complex question, but it really boils down to everybody adhering to a commonly-agreed set of behaviours. If somebody starts to scream, shout, rage, or bully someone, that individual who is being bullied has an immediate recourse because there is a mechanism for him to go to the second-level superior or with HR support and say, *Look, this is what happened on XYZ day. It is not acceptable. It is counter to the agreed behaviours we're all meant to live by and work towards living to every single day, and therefore this guy needs help.*

And I think that's the approach that needs to happen. It's what the Americans call intervention. I worked for an American bank where there was the sort of classic alpha-male toxic individual and eventually, his senior colleagues intervened, and he was sent off to do anger management courses and various other interventions designed to help him so that in turn it would help the team. I think it all starts with a conscious realization that how we behave impacts other people and that if you behave in a way that is not in accordance with a company's desired behaviours, then you will be sat down, and you will be helped. And if you refuse the help, well, you can leave. And if you're given help, you will be expected to change your attitude and behaviour. And I think there need to be those very tough conversations. In the real world, of course, seniority, ego, and revenue-generation get in the way. They are often the excuse for just accepting things as they are, and for accepting an individual's behaviour as it is, not as what it should be. But I don't think that that is sufficient any more.

I've been in the workforce now for over forty years. When I joined the workforce, particularly young employees, junior employees; we had very few rights. And we didn't expect to have any, because the idea was that you got more rights as you got more senior, as you got more valuable to the organization. But people who get senior are not necessarily the best people to be managers or leaders. Often it's because they perform well in a particular role and are then promoted. That does not necessarily mean they have the skills and capabilities to perform in that promoted role. And the organization did not enable them with those skills.

They just assumed that they would be all right, and it still goes on today. People are promoted because they are good salespeople, for example, and suddenly they become area sales managers or a regional sales managers, but they have no idea how to manage or lead people. And the organization expects them to learn through a process of osmosis, which of course doesn't work! The point I'm trying to make is that the organizations need to be much more intentional in thinking about what are the desired behaviours and what are the desired outcomes we all want? What do we need, to enable people to get to those desired outcomes? And I fully accept the point that the bullies need as much as the bullied. Clearly.

BEING ACTIVE PARTICIPANTS IN SETTING FIRM BOUNDARIES AND AGREEMENTS

MK

This is very solid. I like how you talked about making agreements as a team, making agreements within an organization, a set of conduct, those kinds of rules. What are the long-term benefits of setting very clear agreements? Agreements are like boundaries.

Victor

I think the agreement on what are the expected behaviours that everybody has to consistently strive to live up to needs to first be agreed by everyone. And everybody will realize that each individual, not the boss, not HR[109], not their supervisors, not their people manager, but they themselves as well as everybody else needs to live up to them. This is a big jump in the corporate world because the corporate world is full of organizations that are very hierarchical, and people at the base of the pyramid feel they have no real say over anything, and therefore they are

[109] HR: Human Resources

passive observers. And what I'm contending is that they need to be active participants in the co-creation and co-sustaining of the enabling positive workplace culture so that they can excel both as people and as contributors to the business they're working with and for. And that's the big jump; it's almost as big a jump as getting boards of companies to consciously spend time and think about, together with senior management, what are the values we want to live up to? What are the behaviours that will demonstrate those values? These are two big, big, big mindset jumps. But I don't think it's impossible because I really believe younger people today, and people entering the workforce today, will simply not tolerate the kind of treatment that I tolerated because I felt I had no choice. It was either stay and enjoy the benefits of a well-paid job, or go and find something else. There was no sort of mechanism to hold accountable people who were behaving badly because they were senior people, because they were big revenue-generators, or because they were part of the political inner circle. And I think that is what businesses need to do. It's a huge mindset change. And the realization that when somebody breaks a leg, they need time to recover. If somebody has a mental breakdown due to stress imposed on them, or their inability to cope with that stress, they also need time to recover. And I think that message has finally gotten through, certainly to many larger organizations. But it's something that each company needs to consciously think about. To me, it just makes the world a better place. It will certainly make the working world a better place. And it would have the knock-on benefit of having a happier home life. Because if you're unhappy at your job, whether you like it or not, that unhappiness will flow into your private life at home. And that can cause all sorts of other problems. And that sort of linkage between what sort of workplace you've got and your success as an employee, as a contributor at that workplace, and also whether you work for an organization with a positive workplace culture, is what will make your home life happier. If you multiply that, you've got a better society, because each one of us is part of society.

MK

You just answered one more question that I wanted to ask you regarding how individuals can keep themselves in check, whether they are aligned with what they are doing to the organization itself.

Victor

Yeah, it's having the values and then making sure that there are penalties for non-compliance. We humans will only respect the fact that yes, we all know how we should behave, but if there's no consequence for behaving badly, we'll just do what we want. And that's why we need penalties, because it causes individuals to pause and think, well if I do that, there will be consequences for me. And I think that is why it's so critical that when you have the values and you have the penalties for non-compliance, people in the organization have to see that the penalties are enforced when somebody doesn't live up to and practise those values and demonstrate them. And I think that is something that builds trust, and then people will say everybody is being held to the same level of accountability. It doesn't matter whether it's the senior vice president of the organization or one of the more junior executives. I think that is critical—the fact that we're all equally able to behave better and we're all equally able to behave badly if given the opportunity. What I'm arguing for is that we should remove that opportunity.

[laughter]

We should remove that opportunity in the interest of everybody's physical and mental wellbeing and in the interests of really sustaining businesses that can focus on the more important things which are how you serve your customers with greater excellence, what products and services do those customers need, and how you deliver them. I think that should be the focus of every organization, not the ego of a division manager or a CEO.

MK

Very interesting. I think this is solid. Is there anything you would like to say as last words to people who might be reading this book for mental wellness?

Victor

I suppose the advice is always to realize that each of us has an impact, whether we're aware of it or not and to be conscious of our impact on others. What we do, what we say, how we behave, how we treat people, have a direct impact on how they feel and their health. And I think we need to be much more conscious about how we do that. I mean, we've only got to look at the ghastly invasion of Ukraine to understand the impact and result. It's incredible. It's incredible that it's happening at all, but it just shows you what somebody can do when they have all the levers and the big weapons. I think that's the word. We have to realize that we're part of a community and we're all imperfect humans. That's the equality factor. It doesn't matter what your education is, what your socio-economic strata is, where you live, what you drive, what you wear on your wrist . . . none of that matters. What matters is how you treat other human beings. And we need to get back as a society, as a human race, to realizing that we all have an impact on others. And we need to be much more intentional about thinking about it and treating people as we would like to be treated. I think that is the key for all of us.

MK

That was excellent. How are you feeling right now, after the sharing?

Victor

I'm fine, because I have come a long way as an individual and I've had all the ups and downs that anybody and everybody has in life. And from each of them you do learn something. If you want to. And I've always striven to learn something from whatever happens and try then and not replicate the same mistake. I still make mistakes and I will continue to do so because I am an imperfect human being, but I try very hard very consciously to learn from experiences and then take a different approach if I face a similar set of circumstances or issues next time round. That's what I try to do. I don't always succeed, but I try to do it.

MK

I'm learning a lot from this conversation as well, and I think that whatever you just shared is aligned with what I have towards these principles I have. I try to uphold these principles in any of the projects I undertake in my life. I think it's important.

Victor

It's very important. It's part of trust-building. It's part of integrity. It's part of relationship-building. You see, I think that's the other problem: it's very obvious in Singapore that everything has become a transaction. We're a very transactional society. A lot of things are touch-and-go, but in fact that is not what leads to a healthy mental state or good human-to-human relations. Relationships take time. You have to build them. You have to invest energy and time into building and sustaining them. They don't happen overnight and I think that is something we as humans need to understand more. We need to place more value on relationships and much less value on transactions. I think there are signs through this pandemic that many humans are what I call growing up and realizing, particularly when it comes to the equal importance of mental wellbeing to physical health. The two in fact are completely intertwined. And that gives me some optimism, that humans can progress despite the regressive behaviour we're now seeing in Ukraine. But humans can progress if we want to. And I hope it's not a flash in the pan because we're wired to forget: that's how we survive. I just hope that we don't forget the lessons of COVID-19. I hope that we learn those lessons and we practice the positive outcomes from those lessons and continue to progress. There is a lot of evidence around the world that humans are regressing. Whether it's the polarization you see in America and in other countries where you're either with us or against us, and if you're against us you're inherently evil. I mean this is sort of medieval thinking that should have no place in the modern world, but it just shows you how human beings react and respond to the different stimuli and the different influences and how we're all very easily swayed by whatever is populist. Because we gravitate towards easy solutions. Building a positive workplace culture in a company is not easy. And like anything in life that's worth having or worth doing, it takes effort, from all sides—leadership at every level, self-leadership from every employee, and active participation from everyone. It's not easy.

MK

Victor, thank you so much for your time today. This is a very powerful conversation. I really hope that what you just shared will push a lot of people forward into looking into this area, as a responsibility, as a manager, a leader, or even as a staff. We are all responsible for our mental health.

CHAPTER 21

Building a Society That is Forgiving and Forbearing

By John Wong Chee Meng, Senior Consultant Psychiatrist at the Department of Psychological Medicine at the National University Hospital (NUH)

Mental health is a global issue, and there is no simple solution for it. There are a few moving pieces that Dr John Wong Chee Meng shares in his interview. The first is awareness, to encourage individuals to be responsible for their mental wellbeing and emotional wellbeing. The second is for individuals to be aware or mindful of the interaction between oneself and the community, and the third is to cultivate a society that is forbearing and forgiving, and that is a national conversation that calls for a systemic approach to have policies and initiatives that allow these values to thrive.

THERE'S NO PHYSICAL HEALTH WITHOUT MENTAL HEALTH, AND NO MENTAL HEALTH WITHOUT PHYSICAL HEALTH

MK

Could you share more about your professional journey in mental health?

Dr Wong

My professional journey in mental health services started from the very first day I was posted to the old Woodbridge Hospital as a medical student, where we learnt to interview patients in the psychiatric wards. We learnt from the patients who were admitted for their psychological and emotional distress, and most importantly, we learnt from the psychiatric nurses, doctors, and the mental health allied professionals, how they assess, manage, and treat patients who were admitted into Woodbridge Hospital in the 1980s. At that time, Woodbridge Hospital was frequently seen by the public as an asylum, even though it was already providing modernized medical psychiatric treatment and structured vocational rehabilitation services for patients with chronic schizophrenia. Mental healthcare in the early 1980s then focused on providing medication, medical care, assessment, as well as long stay for mental health patients who were rejected by their families or communities. It was an eye-opener as a final-year medical student. But the real exposure to the mental health journey as a working mental health professional came when I finished my housemanship, where seven of us were assigned by the Ministry of Health to serve about six to seven months of medical officer posting in Woodbridge Hospital. We were trained in psychiatry so that when we returned and served our national service in the SAF[110], we could contribute to providing primary psychiatric assessment and care of our soldiers there. And that was the very first immersion experience I had working in a full-fledged mental health hospital in Singapore. Those seven months were a long journey. It opened up my eyes to the challenges of the various mental health conditions, how they are inflicted on individuals, families, society, and how many of them were rejected by some of their family members and had nowhere to turn to, and as a result, had to stay in a hospital. At that time, there were limited opportunities and programmes developed for long-stay patients who were essentially rehabilitated but had no accommodation.

The range of mental health challenges inflicted on the many people who were patients and ex-patients of Woodbridge Hospital was an eye-opener, and that made many of our doctors who worked there realize that we treated physically unwell patients and helped them recover, so that they could return to their family, return to their community, to their workplace, continue to function, and that helped them get accepted back. But for many of our mental health patients with serious co-morbid medical conditions like schizophrenia, psychosis, prolonged alcohol abuse, or those with associated forensic mental health issues, they had a very trying journey in returning to the community. At that time, the stigma of social rejection was very real, and a lot of effort was put in by the ministry and hospital to address that. They worked very hard to have a team of dedicated medical social workers specializing in psychiatric care to investigate how these patients and families could be supported. Those days taught us important lessons that there's no physical health without mental health, and there is also no mental health if they do not have physical health. That was a very important immersion experience for me as a young doctor.

[110] SAF: Singapore Armed Forces

When I returned to serve my National Service, I felt inspired and motivated to want to spend the first part of my career serving the military, and I had various interests in pursuing further training in my medical career. Among the areas of interest were surgical discipline, orthopaedics, and obstetrics, but I soon realized there were many needs in the local mental health service development, both in peacetime and in emergency operations. And that inspired and challenged me to consider spending my first career as a military doctor with a specialization in psychiatry. That was not an easy decision, but it was a decision that inspired me to commit fifteen years of my first career doing mental health and psychiatry in the military, both providing peacetime health care and planning for times of emergency for our soldiers and seamen. It was a very exciting time when I was assigned to serve my first career in SAF as a military psychiatrist and that provided me with the training opportunities to further specialize in trauma psychiatry, where we learnt about mental health management in disaster psychiatry, acute stress, and post-traumatic stress disorders, especially in the context of supporting soldiers and commanders both during training incidents, as well as in operational matters. This helped shape a new perspective in me, that even a very well-equipped individual, when subjected to exceptional situations and stresses in their lifetime, needs to be resilient.

One can be easily overwhelmed by stress from trauma, be it a man-made disaster or natural disaster. That was another important chapter for career learning in mental health. During that time, as part of our services to medical peers, healthcare professionals, and laypeople in educational training, it was really important to gain exposure to clinical and operational research as well as exposure to the teachings of medical students, medics, and laypeople. We were able to see that there's so much to be done, because the mental health literacy at that point in time was very minimal across the population and community.

This opened up the next chapter where we looked at how we could best develop a new area of work in preventive mental health besides treating those who are acutely ill or chronically sick with mental health conditions. At that time, across both the Ministry of Defence (MINDEF) and Ministry of Health, there was great emphasis on many programmes advocating a healthy lifestyle among Singaporeans and the community. We had many programmes that advocated mental health resilience and mental health strength training. These were very important early introductions to preventive mental healthcare, besides caring for those who are unwell. And it's the preventive mental health work that further shaped my career direction, with the organizational commitment in the SAF and MINDEF to train a new group of military psychiatrists to look at how we could better understand the psychopathology and developmental psychology of our Singaporean children who were growing up into their adolescent years before they became young able men and women. And many of them would serve their National Service. It was this early upstream programme that continued to inspire many of us to investigate how best to design this preventive work.

RESTORING FUNCTION IN OCCUPATIONAL, EDUCATIONAL, SOCIAL, AND FINANCIAL ROLES

MK

Got it. What are some of these stigmas that you've observed in your profession, and how do we address them?

Dr Wong

The mental health stigma that we commonly read about in the papers manifests in a couple of ways. One would associate people with mental illness and stigmatize people who appear to have 'lost their minds', or exhibit irrational, strange, disruptive, hostile, or aggressive behaviours, which causes them to stand out in the eyes of the public, thus losing their ability to study, work or socialize. The stigma is further entrenched when they become unwilling to seek professional assessment and help, which compounds their social difficulties. These factors could portray the ill person as socially unreasonable and incapable of becoming well again. This makes people afraid of being identified and labelled with a mental health condition.

More importantly, I believe that stigma, when coming from the community, family members, and medical professionals, is often hard to bear.

In the community, when individuals become unwell, they could be presenting disruptive behaviour at home, at their workplace, or even at their schools, which often alarms people around them—their family members, neighbours, peers, or workplace colleagues. These individuals could also be patients with chronic mental health issues presenting with acute disturbances, manifesting disruptive behaviour in the community they live in.

It is true that a person with acute mental health distress may lose control over themselves emotively or behaviourally, for a moment, or over a period of time. People tend to remember these critical incidents or moments, and the visual memory of the behavioural distress and disruption seems to describe and represent the person from then. Many people do not have the opportunity to see someone recover from a transient illness and return to what they used to be; we call it the pre-morbid personality, or the normal self. As mental health professionals, we have the privilege of witnessing the recovery journey of many patients and seeing how they return to function and return to wellness. This gives us the confidence to want to work in this area and continue the important work of helping more patients or people in distress.

To address the stigmatization of mental illness in today's context, I would say that it's important to first frame stigma differently.

Stigmatization is often associated with acute disruptive behaviour, loss of control, and violence. Stigmatization is often associated with a person who has lost their earning capacity, lost their job, or lost their ability to study. Stigmatization is often associated with the person being left alone to agonize—isolated away from the community or their family. And this so-called 'asocial', or 'anti-social' presentation adds a lot to stigmatization as well.

I would say that fighting against labelling, fighting against hiding one's mental health history, and 'coming out' to share their mental health vulnerabilities with others . . . all this helps. But it would not be enough to destigmatize mental illness, as this does not give a full understanding of what stigmatization is about.

The need to remove society's stigmatization of mental illness is clear. In recent years, it has been actively promoted and advocated by various ministries and agencies. I think they've made good progress. And we have had many luminaries and people coming forth as advocates, as people who have gone through their own mental health struggles. And these celebrities help to bring cheers to the community, reminding us that everyone is vulnerable.

But I think what is more pertinent and more defining in removing stigmatization has to be addressing the root cause. How do we help individuals recover and return to function? If we can help every individual who has a temporary or transient distress, or has a major acute illness or major chronic illness, to recover fully, or partially, and be rehabilitated or restored to a level where the person can restore his function in terms of social, work, earning capacity and ability; where a student is able to return to class, learn, and complete the education programme; where the person can fulfil some of the social roles and expectations from the family, or the community; that's when we can begin removing stigmatization. Unless we address the need to restore function in occupational, educational, social, and financial roles, we will never be able to fully eradicate the notion of stigmatization, because society will still perceive that the individual is not able to contribute and is still different from the person that he or she was.

I would say that stigmatization is a complex and important domain to address in the whole approach of mental health wellness and promotion in society, and it should go beyond getting celebrities and luminaries to come forward to say, *I had this condition.* More importantly, it is for the members of the public and family members to see that we are actively working to help these individuals who may be acutely distressed, chronically distressed, or temporarily distressed to restore some—if not all—their functions across the domains mentioned earlier, and for them to value the individuals in the state that they are in. I think that is the day that we will remove the stigmatization of mental illness.

MK

Got it.

Dr Wong

Whatever we see and hear in the media helps to raise mental health literacy. Raising mental health awareness and advocating for mental wellness is essential, but the full work must include restoring function.

PLANTING TREES WHOSE SHADE WE KNOW WE MAY NOT SIT IN

MK

Just now, you actually mapped out the different causes and effects of the stigmas around mental health. I'm just wondering, as an intervention, what can an individual do at a personal level, to make sure that their own mental health is taken care of and is strengthened? What can we do as a community collectively, so that we can bring all these people together to create an ecosystem that supports people in the resolution of their mental health struggles?

Dr Wong

I think this is a very global issue. There's no simple solution to this, but I can see a few moving pieces that will contribute towards solving the puzzle.

One is that if we want to achieve or encourage individuals to be responsible for their mental wellbeing and emotional wellbeing, the first step is awareness. So mental health literacy is important. It's just like being aware that high blood sugar levels can bring us diabetes, and diabetes can cause blood vessel and tissue injuries and increase the risk of end-organ injury. Poor wound-healing could increase the risk of developing gangrene in the limbs, leading to their amputation in severe cases, or we may even end up with end-stage renal failure after many years of poor diabetic control. Unless you are aware, you will not even contemplate taking preventive action and adopting a healthy lifestyle. Awareness through increased literacy is probably the very first important step at the individual level.

The second is for the individual to be aware or be mindful of the interaction between oneself and the community that we belong to. It is important to have an understanding of one's temperament, personality, strength and resilience, and the constitution within us in terms of our own emotional or psychological makeup. Some of us can be a little bit more emotive, while some are a little bit more detached. Some of us actually may have some genetic risks that, when interacting with disadvantageous environmental factors, could place us at greater risk of developing certain major mental health conditions like schizophrenia, depression, anxiety, autism, ADHD[111], and so on. While having the genetic risk doesn't mean that we will develop it, by just knowing that there's a risk, we can actively keep ourselves well by adopting strategies and life skills to mitigate and lower the risk. This is no different from having grandparents and parents with diabetes mellitus and the person saying, *Okay, I'll be very careful with my caloric intake, I'll be very careful with my exercise, I'll be very careful with my BMI*, and choosing to stay active in exercise and adopt a healthy diet as early as possible—in their teenage and young adult years. Then the individuals running the risk of developing diabetes will be lower, or they might delay the onset till much later, or hopefully avoid even developing diabetes in old age. While the risk is there, it can be contained, delayed, or mitigated. In the same light, for people with a family history of certain major psychiatric or mental health conditions, we need not despair. We should be cognizant of it, recognize that there's a risk, and look at ways to keep ourselves well mentally and emotionally, and recognize the early symptoms so that we get early help, early intervention, and receive early treatment should some of these symptoms surface along the way.

In public health strategies, there are three levels of illness prevention. The first level is primary prevention—to prevent it from happening. The second level of prevention is where if a condition does develop, then early detection and early treatment of the individual allows for recovery, and they need not suffer any long-term consequences. Tertiary prevention is when it has already happened, when complications are starting to happen, but we intervene so that the individual does not develop full-blown injuries or serious consequences. For example, somebody who already has diabetes for years may start to develop eye changes or kidney changes. Then the tertiary prevention would entail

[111] ADHD: Attention Deficit Hyperactivity Disorder

the individual to very close kidney care and eye care to delay the deterioration of the kidney and eye function. So mental health prevention strategies are no different from physical health prevention strategies.

At the community level, it is important to look at creating an ecosystem system for mental wellness. Two things would come to mind. One is to be forgiving and forbearing. In today's terms, it is to create an inclusive society. How we arrive there, to develop an inclusive society that is forgiving and forbearing—that is altogether another national conversation! Essentially, the spirit of an inclusive society is reflected in our day-to-day lives, in how the social-financial-political ecosystem supports and accommodates ethnic minorities, offers equal opportunity, in how we treat foreign workers, and so on. It boils down to building an inclusive society that is forbearing and forgiving.

How to be forbearing and forgiving? Not many people can do that. There are incident reports in newspapers from time to time that alert us to these potential fault lines. We have to look from a systemic approach: What are our social values, physical environments, and policies, that would allow us to support the building of an inclusive, forgiving, forbearing society? More importantly, some of us would ask: *If we have a forgiving, forbearing society, would there be people who would take advantage of, cannibalize, and abuse the system?* Again, this is another interesting mindset that, as a larger ecosystem, we have to address. One example is when we look at our physical house and environment. In our HDB[112] flats, apartments, and houses, we install security grills with locks. But when you watch Hollywood movies and visit friends living in the secured suburbs of some Western countries, you realize that sometimes they leave their keys underneath the doormat. Sometimes the doors are not locked. To us, they're foolish and

[112] HDB: Housing Development Board (public housing in Singapore)

too trusting. For Asians, we talk about crime prevention. We talk about being careful, diligent, and astute. I guess the whole idea is about how we can calibrate a society that is trusting enough that you don't have to be too suspicious of people pilfering or taking advantage of the system, versus a situation where everything must be under lock and key and constantly watched under CCTV. I applaud many of our community Mayors and Grassroots Advisors and MPs[113]. For example when they trial ran umbrella sharing programmes in neighbourhoods, where they put umbrellas at the corner of bus stops. People take one when it's raining, and when they are finished with it, they return it. I applaud the few initiatives of setting up the void deck foodbank, where people are encouraged to share fresh food by leaving them in the foodbank fridges. This is a good start.

MK

Yes, the communal fridges.

Dr Wong

And people can put in food, and you just take what you need. It does take generations to evolve the give-and-take spirit—normally known as kampong spirit! We may have lost it somewhat, but we can work to build up again in our generation. In the meantime, there may be a small number of people who take advantage of the system, but the success of all these schemes is not to be measured by whether people are doing it now. Rather, I would suggest that success be defined as when the children and grandchildren of the current generation develop this kampong spirit and value system and live out the behaviour as advocated by such schemes. We should look at building an inclusive, forgiving,

---

[113] MP: Member of Parliament

and forbearing society not expecting a complete change during our generation, but expecting that the values and ideas will be seeded into the children and grandchildren of our generation, and that these value systems will be their norm when they grow up to be adults.

I would say that whatever we do today to advocate mental health, wellness, and destigmatization, it's important to start now. But we also must be cognizant that when we plant a tree today, its shade may only come in the next generation. But if you don't plant a tree today, there will never be any shade for the next generation. We just need to be patient ourselves. If it brings about shade to enjoy, with an earlier change of the value system and practices of people, I think it will be a bonus. If it does not happen in our generation but shows evidence of it happening in the next two generations, it will still be a deserving effort and needs to be done.

The path to finding the answers is not easy by any means, and sometimes the answers aren't what we expect them to be. But there are 1,001 reasons not to do something, and you only need one to do it—because **your life matters.** Doors and windows of opportunity open when they do, and it is up to you to step in. If the experience of this book has sparked something deeper in you that you wish to examine, let this be another sign from the universe to keep going.

If you'd like to reach out to have a conversation with us, our doors are open.

Send us a message on Instagram at **@thisconnect.today,** and we'll be happy to connect with you.

Bibliography

Newman, Alexander, Ross Donohue and Nathan Eva, 'Psychological safety: A systematic review of the literature.' *Human Resource Management Review* 27, 3 (2017): 521–535, https://doi.org/10.1016/j.hrmr.2017.01.001

Seow, Bei Yi 'A black plaster, to talk about feelings.' *The Straits Times,* 2011, https://www.straitstimes.com/singapore/health/a-black-plaster-to-talk-about-feelings

Deci, Edward L. and Richard M. Ryan, 'Self-determination theory,' *Handbook of Theories of Social Psychology* 1, (2012): 416–436, https://doi.org/10.4135/9781446249215.n21

Jovanovic, Dragana, and Marina Matejevic, 'Relationship between Rewards and Intrinsic Motivation for Learning - Researches Review.' *Procedia - Social and Behavioral Sciences* 149, 5 (2014): 456–460, https://doi.org/10.1016/j.sbspro.2014.08.287

Economist Intelligence Unit, 'Worldwide Cost of Living 2020.' https://www.eiu.com/n/campaigns/worldwide-cost-of-living-2020.

Ozbay, Faith et al., 'Social Support and Resilience to Stress.' *Psychiatry* (Edgmont) 4, 5 (2007), 35–40, https://www.ncbi.nlm.nih.gov/pmc/articles/PMC2921311/

Giorgi, Gabriele et al., 'COVID-19-Related Mental Health Effects in the Workplace: A Narrative Review.' *Int J Environ Res Public*

Health 17, 21 (2020), 7857, https://pubmed.ncbi.nlm.nih.gov/33120930/

Gallup, 'Item 3: Doing What I Do Best.' *Gallup,* 1999, https://www.gallup.com/workplace/237542/item-doing-best.aspx

Yaribeygi, Habib et al., 'The Impact of Stress on Body Function: A Review.' *EXCLI Journal 16,* (2017), 1057–1072, doi: 10.17179/excli2017-480

Khoo, Leslie, 'Singapore Healthcare Market-Share Analysis.' *Ministry of Health,* 2003, https://www.moh.gov.sg/docs/librariesprovider5/resources-statistics/information-papers/singapore_healthcare_market-share_analysis.pdf

Kurohi, Rei, 'New task force to tackle mental health needs of Singaporeans amid pandemic.' *The Straits Times*, 2020, https://www.straitstimes.com/singapore/health/task-force-to-tackle-mental-health-needs-amid-pandemic

Eisma, Maarten C., Paul A. Boelen and Lonneke I.M. Lenferink, 'Prolonged grief disorder following the Coronavirus (COVID-19) pandemic.' *Psychiatry Res* 288, 113031 (2020), https://doi.org/10.1016/j.psychres.2020.113031

Ministry of Health, 'Percentage of Spending on Mental Health, Diabetes and Ageing Versus Total Healthcare Spending in 2018 Against Amount Budgeted for 2019.' https://www.moh.gov.sg/news-highlights/details/percentage-of-spending-on-mental-health-diabetes-and-ageing-versus-total-healthcare-spending-in-2018-against-amount-budgeted-for-2019/

Moss, Jennifer, 'Beyond Burned Out.' *Harvard Business Review,* 2021, https://hbr.org/2021/02/beyond-burned-out.

Oh, Tessa, 'Review of Singapore's Mental Healthcare System Underway, as MPs Highlight Existing Gaps.' *TODAYonline,* 2020, https://www.todayonline.com/singapore/review-singapores-mental-healthcare-system-underway-mps-highlight-existing-gaps

V. Stefanoudis, Paris, et al., 'Turning the tide of parachute science.' *Current Biology* 31, no. 4 (2021): R184–R185, https://doi.org/10.1016/j.cub.2021.01.029

Subramaniam, M., E. Abdin, J. A. Vaingankar, S. Shafie, B.Y. Chua, R. Sambasivam, Y. J. Zhang, et al., 'Tracking the Mental Health of a Nation: Prevalence and Correlates of Mental Disorders in the Second Singapore Mental Health Study.' *Epidemiology and Psychiatric Sciences* 29, 2020: e29, doi:10.1017/S2045796019000179.

Tan, Theresa, 'S'pore landmark study finds children of convicted offenders more likely to get into trouble with the law.' *The Straits Times*, 2021, https://www.straitstimes.com/singapore/spore-landmark-study-finds-children-of-convicted-offenders-more-likely-to-get-into-trouble

Theseira, Walter, 'What Are The Demographics Of Patients Receiving Psychiatric Treatment And Mental Health Support.' *Ministry of Health*, 2020, https://www.moh.gov.sg/news-highlights/details/what-are-the-demographics-of-patients-receiving-psychiatric-treatment-and-mental-health-support.

Acknowledgements

I would like to express our heartfelt gratitude to all the people who have played a part in making this book come to life. To our contributors, thank you for jumping in and contributing your time, energy, and intention towards forwarding the mental health scene in Singapore. It is a work in progress, and perhaps it may take more than just one lifetime to see the transformation unfold, yet your desire to make a difference to the people out there is instrumental to keeping the vision alive for our future generations, in wellness and prosperity. I am grateful to all of you for the good work that is being done out there and I look forward to more efficient and effective interventions to touch the lives out there.

To the people working with me in the background, Si Qi and Megan, I want to thank you for supporting me in facilitating the process so that these interviews and the backend work could happen. Your beliefs in the cause and my vision, your stand, dedication, and devotion in the project have inspired me to keep going, to push forth to produce a higher quality of work that is nothing less than being impeccable and excellent. This book would not have been completed without your support and commitment.

We embarked on this project with the simple objective to document the different perspectives around mental health in Singapore, yet we walked out of each interview session feeling deeply inspired by selfless acts of service from all these contributors. These interview sessions have shaped our understanding of what service to the community means, no matter big or small, and we deeply cherish the life lessons and personal takeaways we received from all the contributors.

I would also like to attribute and honor all my masters and teachers for being my greatest sources of inspiration for my work, and the trust and faith they placed in me in carrying the work forward to make a difference in this world; trusting in me to do the right thing and getting my act together during my lowest point and being there with me to celebrate my successes and endeavors during my highest peaks. Without them, I would not have been the person I am today. Every single day, I wake up looking forward to live my mark with love, passion and joy.

Finally, I would like to conclude with a quote from Thoreau, Henry David Thoreau, *Walden, or Life in the Woods*:

'I went to the woods because I wished to live deliberately, to front only the essential facts of life, and see if I could not learn what it had to teach, and not, when I came to die, discover that I had not lived. I did not wish to live what was not life, living is so dear; nor did I wish to practice resignation, unless it was quite necessary. I wanted to live deep and suck out all the marrow of life, to live so sturdily and Spartan-like as to put to rout all that was not life, to cut a broad swath and shave close, to drive life into a corner, and reduce it to its lowest terms, and, if it proved to be mean, why then to get the whole and genuine meanness of it, and publish its meanness to the world; or if it were sublime, to know it by experience, and be able to give a true account of it in my next excursion.'

This is an experience we will remember for a lifetime, and we hope that it has inspired you to continue doing the work that you do too. This is only the beginning, and there is so much more to learn, many more steps to take, and much more work to be done. We hope to honour all our contributors by doing our part to champion mental health causes so that we can create an inclusive, thriving society where people are deeply connected to themselves, to the present, and to the world around them. Thank you.

Acknowledgements

Adrian Pang
Pangdemonium

Amirah Munawwarah
ImPossible Psychological Services

Andrea Chan
Joel Wong
Lucia Chow
Peggy Lim
TOUCH Community Services Ltd

Asher Low
Limitless

Belinda Ang
ARTO by thinkART of the Box Pte Ltd

Brenda Lee
Lynn Tan
The Psychology Practice

Buvenasvari Pragasam
Solace Art Psychotherapy Pte Ltd

Camellia Wong
InPsychful LLP

Carrie Tan
Nee Soon South (Nee Soon GRC)

Calvin Eng
Association for Music Therapy (Singapore)

Charlotte Goh
Playeum

Cheryl Chan
Fengshan (East Coast GRC)

Cayden Woo
Jeremy Heng
Singapore Children's Society

Cho Ming Xiu
Campus PSY Limited

Daphne Chua
Somatic Therapy Asia

David Chew
National Heritage Board

David Lim
Tzu Chi Free Clinic
Special Oral Care Network

Deborah Seah
Nadera Binte Abdul Aziz
Community of Peer Support Specialists (CPSS)

Desmond Chew
Jacqueline
Jamie
Mysara
Caregivers Alliance Limited

Desmond Soh
Annabelle Psychology

Eric Chua
Ministry of Culture, Community and Youth
Ministry of Social and Family Development

Etsegenet Mulugeta Eshete
Margaret Hoffer
Selamta Family Project

Goh Li Shan
REACH (West)
Department of Psychological Medicine, National University Hospital

Hannah Batrisyia
Muhammad Syazan Bin Saad
Temasek Polytechnic

Jamus Lim
Anchorvale (Sengkang GRC)

Jasmine Yeo
The Private Practice

Jenny Ng
Conscious Parenting Coach
(MEd of Family Education)

Jingzhou
Cassia Resettlement Team

Josephine Chia-Teo
InSightful Training & Consultancy Pte Ltd

John Wong Chee Meng
Department of Psychological Medicine, National University Hospital

Jun Lee
Self-employed Art Therapist and Art Facilitator

Karen Wee
Lions Befrienders Service Association

Kyl Lim
Singapore Cancer Society

Lynette Har
ICF-Certified Peak Performance Coach

Lynette Seow
Safe Space™

Marion Neubronner
Psychologist and Leadership Development Coach

Michelle Koay
St. Joseph's Institution International Ltd

Murali Pillai
Bukit Batok SMC

Narasimman S/O Tivasiha Mani
Impart Ltd

Navin Amarasuriya
The Contentment Foundation

Natalie Kang
Art for Good Pte Ltd
MySpace Psychotherapy Services Pte Ltd

Nicole K.
The Tapestry Project SG

Jolene
Volunteer in the Migrant Workers' Space

Nur Farhan Bte Mohammad Alami
Raffles Medical Group

Ng Gim Choo
The EtonHouse Group
Ng Jek Mui
Dementia Singapore

(formerly known as Alzheimer's Disease Association)

Patrick Tay
Pioneer SMC

Rachel Yang
Daylight Creative Therapies

Ronald P.M.H. Lay
LASALLE College of the Arts

Roshni Bhatia
Yoko Choi
FoundSpace

Seah Kian Peng
Braddell Heights (Marine Parade GRC)

Serene Seng
Senserene Pte Ltd

Siew Kum Yew
Shan You Counselling Centre

Simone Heng
Human Connection Speaker

Sujata Tiwari
CEO of HMZ

Sun Kaiying
Hope for Tomorrow Psychology Centre

Sufian Yusof
Aileron Wellness

Tina Hung
National Council of Social Service (NCSS)

Tin Pei Ling
MacPherson SMC

Wan Rizal Bin Wan Zakariah
Kolam Ayer (Jalan Besar GRC)

Vickineswarie Jagadharan
OTHERS

Victor Mills
Michael Chang

Singapore International Chamber of Commerce

Ying Jie

About THISCONNECT.TODAY

THIS
. CON
NECT

ThisConnect is a mental health advocacy community set up to spark more conscious awareness and forwarding interventions on mental health, emotional wellness, and suicide prevention using experiential art. We recognise the need to begin the mental health conversations by examining the personal struggles that weigh us down in life. These everyday stressors can seem insignificant on their own, but over a long period of time, they can make us feel trapped, lost, stressed, and depressed. Through our work, we want to inspire more people to step out, to connect consciously and deeply with themselves physically, emotionally, mentally and spiritually, and to find the healing with the good and the bad, the positive and the negative, the light and the shadow within them. We want people to access their courage, love, freedom in their beings to express their most authentic selves, and to create a life where they are thriving. We hope that our work will empower individuals to seek help and to look inwards whenever they face challenges in life.

Since 2020, we have presented three large multimedia art exhibitions and thirteen moving satellite shows in Singapore, titled *ThisConnect: Threading Worlds*, Masks of Singapore, and *ThisConnect: What Am I, If I Am Not*, and were featured in *The Straits Times*,

Tatler, Channel 8. Masks of Singapore, a six-month community participatory art project movement, has set the record for the 'Largest Mosaic of Hand-Sculptured Masks' in the Singapore Book of Records and were documented into a photobook with Fujifilm that tells 572 lived-stories of individuals from all walks of lives in their most authentic self behind the masks created.

For more information, reach out at

ThisConnect.today@gmail.com.
https://www.thisconnect.today
https://www.instagram.com/thisconnect.today

'Oftentimes, external expectations about who we should be and how we should act prevent us from being free to express ourselves and do the things that truly matter to us. As a result, many of us end up chasing after societal definitions of success instead of what truly matters to us, and we end up lost, confused, and disconnected from ourselves. It is this disconnection from ourselves that forms the start of the many mental and emotional struggles we face every day, and it is potentially leads to depression, and on a more severe scale, suicide. Through our work, we aim to explore the deeper conversations that underpin the mental health struggles many of us battle in our daily lives and empower people to connect to themselves, to the present, and the world around them. Ultimately, the goal is to see a society where people are free to be bold, be free, and be themselves—unapologetically—so that they can begin to live a life that matters to them.'

Hun Ming Kwang,
Founder, Creative Director,
Author of ThisConnect.today